369 0154484

KU-415-294

F. Stiefel (Ed.)

Communication in Cancer Care

With 6 Figures and 10 Tables

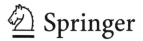 Springer

Prof. Friedrich Stiefel, MD
Médecin Chef de Service
Service de Psychiatrie de Liaison
CHUV
Rue du Bugnon 44
1011 Lausanne
Switzerland

Library of Congress Control Number: 2006920556
ISSN 0080-0015
ISBN 10 3-540-30757-5   Springer Berlin Heidelberg New York
ISBN 13 978-3-540-30757-0   Springer Berlin Heidelberg New York

Springer is a part of Springer Science + Business Media
springeronline.com

© Springer-Verlag Berlin Heidelberg 2006
Printed in Germany

Editor: Dr. Ute Heilmann, Heidelberg
Desk editor: Dörthe Mennecke-Bühler, Heidelberg
Cover design: Frido Steinen Broo, eStudio Calamar, Spain
Production & Typesetting: LE-TeX Jelonek, Schmidt & Vöckler GbR, Leipzig
Printed on acid-free paper   SPIN 11596073   5 4 3 2 1 0

To Fabienne, Axelle and Léa

Foreword

Communication as the Bridge to Hope and Healing in Cancer Care

Cancer is often seen as precipitating an existential crisis; a crisis of spirit and an opportunity for meaning. This is true not only for the patient with cancer and his or her family and loved ones, but also, interestingly enough, for oncologists and cancer care providers. For the patient the challenges are dealing with fear and uncertainty, maintaining a balance between hope and despair, comprehending information and enacting shared decision making, living with choices, and, for too many, finding a way to accept death. For the family the challenges are equally daunting; finding a way to support their loved one and help them maintain hope, advocate on their behalf, help collect and integrate information. This must all be done while not allowing one's own fear and depression to produce a state of isolation for the patient. For the oncologist and other cancer care providers the challenges are fierce as well; finding a way to impart information clearly, finding a way to empower patients in a shared decision making endeavor, finding a way to maintain hope and most importantly somehow finding a way to prevent technology and modern science from dehumanizing the doctor–patient relationship. What we are learning, from this new and rapidly evolving field of cancer communication research and training, is that good communication in cancer care can be a bridge to hope and healing.

Communication issues in cancer care begin even before a cancer diagnosis, in cancer prevention strategies, and extend to all phases of treatment, survivorship and end-of-life care. Communication in cancer care involves the patient and the family, as well as all the members of the cancer treatment team. Finally, communication in cancer care must address issues specific to patients of all ages, diverse cultures and lifestyles. Perhaps two of the most well-developed areas in communication in cancer care relate to shared decision-making research, and the effectiveness of communication skills training of cancer care providers. The field of communication research and training is thus quite broad and still in development, although much has been accomplished, as is illustrated in this textbook.

This text, *Communication in Cancer Care* edited by F. Stiefel, represents one of the most comprehensive as well as clinically relevant edited volumes on the subject of communication in cancer care to appear to date. Professor Stiefel has enlisted international experts in a very broad range of cancer communication areas including: cancer prevention, genetic counseling, all phases of cancer treatment, palliative care, communication with children, families, culturally specific communications, interdisciplinary communication and communication skills training. The table of contents contains some interesting juxtapositions of chapters including a chapter on "Informing About Diagnosis, Relapse and Progression of Disease – Communication with the Terminally Ill Cancer Patient" by Drs. Stiefel and Razavi, followed by a chapter on "Maintaining Hope: Communication in Palliative Care" by Dr. Mary Lloyd Williams.

The contributors include an international array of experts in cancer communication and psycho-oncology. Contributors represent experts from Switzerland, Belgium, England, France, Germany, The Netherlands and Italy. This international perspective is a testament not only to the relevance of cancer communication throughout all cultures, but also to the growing importance and interest of the oncology and psycho-oncology communities in developing research and training in communication in cancer care. This also represents the recognition that the delivery of optimal cancer care cannot take place without skillful, effective, and compassionate communication taking place.

As we face the future of cancer care, it is clear that we are in store for more advances in technology, diagnostics and treatment that have the potential to create an even greater detachment between the patient and the cancer care provider. The potential for further de-humanizing or de-personalizing the practice of oncology is readily evident. Thus the importance of communication in cancer care grows greater and more critically relevant with every passing moment. This text represents a major advance for the field of communication in cancer care, and its publication is timely and well received.

On a personal note, I am particularly gratified that Prof. Stiefel has given me the opportunity to write a few words of introduction to the text he so skillfully created and edited. Our professional relationship and personal friendship dates back almost 20 years, to the period of time that Prof. Stiefel and I conducted our first research studies together at Memorial Sloan-Kettering Cancer Center. It gives me great pleasure to congratulate him on this extraordinary contribution to the fields of Psycho-oncology and Cancer Communication.

William Breitbart, MD, FAPM
Professor and Chief, Psychiatry Service
Memorial Sloan-Kettering Cancer Center
New York, NY, USA

Contents

List of Contributors

Raphaël Bize, MD
Institute for Social and Preventive Medicine
Lausanne University Hospital
rue du Bugnon 44
1011 Lausanne
Switzerland

Anne Brédart, PhD
Psycho-Oncology Unit
Institut Curie
26, rue d'Ulm
75246 Paris cedex 05
France

Jacques Cornuz, Prof., MD, MPH
Department of Internal Medicine/
Institute of Social and Preventive Medicine
Lausanne University Hospital
rue du Bugnon 44
1011 Lausanne
Switzerland

Jean-Nicolas Despland, Prof., MD
Psychotherapy Research Unit
Department of Psychiatry
Lausanne University Hospital
rue du Bugnon 44
1011 Lausanne
Switzerland

Chris De Valck, PhD
University of Hasselt
Faculty of Medicine
Limburg University Centre
Universiteitslaan
3590 Diepenbeek
Belgium

Sylvie Dolbeault, MD
Psycho-Oncology Unit
Institut Curie
26, rue d'Ulm
75248 Paris Cedex 05
France

Lesley Fallowfield, Prof., MD
Cancer Research UK
Psychosocial Oncology Group
Brighton & Sussex Medical School
University of Sussex
Falmer, Brighton
East Sussex, BN1 9QG
UK

Nathalie Favre
Psychiatry Service
Lausanne University Hospital
rue du Bugnon 44
1011 Lausanne
Switzerland

Pam Firth, RN
Head of Family Support
Isabel Hospice
Watchmead
Welwyn Garden City AL7 1LT
UK

Cécile Flahault
Psycho-Oncology Unit
Institut Curie
26, rue d'Ulm
75248 Paris Cedex 05
France

Martha A. Grootenhuis, PhD
Pediatric Psychosocial Department
Emma Children's Hospital
Meibergdreef 9
1105 AZ Amsterdam
The Netherlands

Valerie Jenkins
Cancer Research UK
Psychosocial Oncology Group
Brighton & Sussex Medical School
University of Sussex
Falmer, Brighton
East Sussex, BN1 9QG
UK

Vida Kennedy, BSc
Division of Primary Care
School of Population, Community and
Behavioural Sciences
University of Liverpool
Brownlow Hill
Liverpool L69 3GB
UK

Alexander Kiss, Prof., MD
Universitätsspital Basel
Psychosomatik
Hebelstrasse 2
4031 Basel
Switzerland

Bob. F. Last, PhD
Pediatric Psychosocial Department
Emma Children's Hospital
Meibergdreef 9
1105 AZ Amsterdam
The Netherlands

Mari Lloyd-Williams, MD
Division of Primary Care
School of Population, Community
and Behavioural Sciences
University of Liverpool
Brownlow Hill
Liverpool L69 3GB
UK

Edel Maex, MD
ZNA Middelheim
Lindereef 1
2020 Antwerpen
Belgium

Françoise Porchet, RN
Service de la Formation Continue CHUV
Mont-Paisible 16
1011 Lausanne
Switzerland

Darius Razavi, Prof., MD
Psycho-Oncology, Pain and Treatment and
Palliative Care Clinic
Institut Jules Bordet
121 Boulevard de Waterloo
1000 Brussels
Belgium

Wolfgang Söllner, Prof., MD
Klinik für Psychosomatik und
Psychotherapeutische Medizin
Klinikum Nürnberg
Prof.-Ernst-Nathan-Str. 1
90419 Nürnberg
Germany

Friedrich Stiefel, Prof., MD
Service de Psychiatrie de Liaison
Lausanne University Hospital
rue du Bugnon 44
1011 Lausanne
Switzerland

Dominique Stoppa-Lyonnet, MD, PhD
Genetic Oncology Service
Institut Curie
26, rue d'Ulm
75248 Paris Cedex 05
France

Antonella Surbone, MD, PhD, FACP
Teaching Research Development Department
European School of Oncology
via del Bollo 4
20123 Milan
Italy

1 Key Elements of Communication in Cancer Care

E. Maex, C. De Valck

Recent Results in Cancer Research, Vol. 168
© Springer-Verlag Berlin Heidelberg 2006

Summary

In this chapter the "communication compass" is introduced. It defines the key elements of communication and provides a language with which to communicate about communication in cancer care. The communication compass consists of two axes. One axis defines the associated perspectives of the clinician and the patient, the other axis the content of information and emotional experience.

"Two lovers sat on a park bench with their bodies touching each other, holding hands in the moonlight. There was silence between them. So profound was their love for each other, they needed no words to express it." (Samuel Johnson)

Sometimes communication just flows. There are these special moments, as fleeting as they are intense. Often communication is stuck. It is as if we speak another language and never manage to understand one another. The lovers on the park bench need no words to express what they feel, neither do they need words to speak about communication. Where communication gets stuck, we need a suitable language to speak about communication.

Professional communication cannot be learned from a cookbook. Most of all it implies a readiness to communicate, which means openness to the other. The old adage that it is impossible not to communicate is only true if no criterion of quality is applied. As soon as some mutual understanding is implied in the definition of communication, the fact that it is at all possible to communicate becomes a miracle.

Since there is an important gap between theory and practice, we created a tool that aims to bridge that gap. We call it the communication compass. It does not propose a model of "ideal communication," but provides a language with which to examine and analyze specific situations and to determine what the pitfalls and possibilities are. It is useful as a tool for identifying communicational difficulties in daily clinical practice and it can serve as a model for training basic communication skills (see Fig. 1).

1.1 Communication Compass

1.1.1 Perspectives

"You're lucky," the oncologist tells his patient with breast cancer. "Your tumor seems to respond well to the hormone therapy. And we still have a lot more possibilities in the future." "Does that mean that I am going to be cured after all?" the woman asks. After the consultation the doctor sighs: "How is it possible after all the explanations I have given, that the patient still has not understood that this therapy does not have a curative intent?"

The first axis in the compass is the axis of perspectives. Who is lucky in the above-mentioned example? It is the doctor who is lucky, because his therapy is working. From the perspective of the patient, being lucky has a completely different meaning. She does not know the doctor's other patients. For her, being lucky means to be free of cancer. That is how she understands her doctor's statement. Doctor and patient look at the same situation from a completely different perspective.

Our scientific mind is not familiar with thinking in perspectives. On the contrary, the essence of science is to approach an objective point of view, independent from perspectives. The weight of an object is measured independently of the one who has to carry it. What is heavy for one may be light for another, but expressed in kilograms it is the same for both. In communication, we have little use for this objectivity. Reality is different from a different perspective. Both perspectives are equally important. Perspectives are the raw material of communication.

The first point in communication is the recognition of the perspective of the other. The key question is: what does the world look like through the eyes of my patient? The problem is that we only have access to our own perspective. We are not wired to our patient. We will never know what it is to be him or her. The question remains open, and has to be put over and over again without ever getting a final answer. In Zen there is a saying that when you have not seen someone for more than two minutes, you no longer know him.

The miracle of communication is that without having direct access to the other's perspective, we can have a feeling of mutual understanding. Communication is based on the recognition of two perspectives. That does not mean it always implies agreement. We can achieve mutual understanding and still realize that our experience of the world, our values and beliefs are completely different.

An important caveat here is not to lose sight of your own perspective. This sometimes happens when, with a lot of goodwill, we try to empathize with the perspective of the other and lose ourselves in that perspective, temporarily forgetting our own view. Our patients do not benefit from our absence in the communication process. When either one perspective gets lost, mutual understanding is lost.

1.1.2 Information and Experience

Case 1
- Jansen Maria, 34 years old, married with two children.
- Breast cancer, T1 N3 Mx
- R/radiotherapy

Case 2
- It hasn't quite sunk in. She functions as if intoxicated. Every now and then the harsh reality comes through. Cancer! What about the children now? And my husband? She freezes. It cannot be, it cannot be true.

Both cases above refer to the same patient, at the same moment, but the two descriptions are in no way similar. "Case 1" contains pure information about the patient's medical status. "Case 2" describes her experience. The difference between information and experience is presented here in

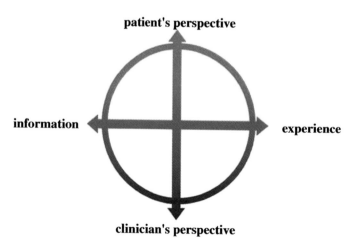

Fig. 1 Communication compass

an extreme way. In communication, both aspects are present at the same time. Therefore, the second axis of the communication compass consists of "information" and "experience." The two aspects of communication must not be confused.

The head nurse notifies the doctor that Mr. Hermans has a request for euthanasia. When the doctor questions him, he is surprised. In a moment of great distress he has exclaimed, "Please let me die, I can stand this no longer." He had never meant this to be taken literally. He does not want to die. Certainly not now, that his new pain medication starts to work.

The typical mistake is that an expression of the patient's ongoing experience (despair) is taken as information (a request for euthanasia). Information and experience are not interchangeable. A request for information should be answered with information, and an expression of experience is to be answered by acknowledging the patient's experience.

Mr. Jones is a retired physician. He is treated for prostate cancer. After his last consultation with the urologist he feels upset. The urologist told him, "According to the statistics of prostate cancer, you still have 13 years to live. According to the statistics for the healthy population you have, 15 years to live."

However correct and reassuring the information may seem to be, it upsets the patient because it ignores his experience of fear. It is erroneous to assume that information counteracts fear. Experience needs recognition. That does not always imply more time. It would have been entirely different for the patient if the doctor had started his sentence with "I understand you are afraid", followed by exactly the same information.

"Doctor, I want to know, is it cancer?" "You don't need to be worried so much. Medicine nowadays has a lot more means than it used to have to cure your condition."

The opposite is a pitfall as well. When asked for information, one should not try to escape delivering bad news by focusing on the emotional experience. Only correct information about diagnosis and possible treatment is the adequate response to this question.

1.1.3 Information

Giving information is challenging. Often we think we have done our job when we have explained it all to the patient, only to be disappointed that he did not understand our explanation. The word "giving" in "giving information" is misleading. When I give you my watch, you have it and I have lost it. When I give you information I do not lose anything, and there is no guarantee that you have it. Information is not something you can "give."

With regard to information, the clinician is in the role of the expert. That is what he has studied for. The patient (usually) does not have that background. The consequence is that the patient receives the information in a very different frame of reference.

It is important to find out what the patient's frame of reference is. How does he perceive his situation? What does he know and how does he understand what he knows? Effective transfer of information starts with probing where the patient is. Assuming that the patient automatically understands the information you give him is a very effective recipe for misunderstanding and frustration (on both sides).

"Let's have a look at the results. The blood tests seem OK and on the scan nothing has changed. Only the result of the pathology test is problematic; it says you have a high grade B-cell lymphoma." "So I don't have cancer after all?"

It is important to present information in a clear, and for the patient understandable, language. Do not, as illustrated above, start with the less important and seemingly reassuring. Do not try to make it feel better than it is. Bad news in inherently bad. Start with what is essential and only then move into details, if the patient still understands you. Then, check how the patient has understood your message. Especially in the case of bad news, the patient may get lost in his experience and no longer hear what you are saying. Often it is necessary to repeat information time after time. Since you never know how the other receives the information, always check.

1.1.4 Experience

John remains in bed the whole day. Lung cancer. He hardly looks up as his wife enters. She has brought his favorite food and his newspaper. She tries to cheer him up. "I'm dying," he says without looking at her. "You have to stay positive," she says, "the doctors are trying their best to help you." He sighs.

In this story the patient's emotional experience is the key element. John does not say much, but his silence speaks louder than words. The tragedy is that it is not heard.

In the domain of personal experience the clinician is no longer the expert. The patient is the expert of his own experience. Consequently it is not the clinician's responsibility to "solve" the patient's experience. This is not easy since we are trained to solve problems. But for John's dying and his sadness there is no solution. Nobody can take away the emotions. They are a natural part of what is going on and there is nothing to solve. Helpers hate being helpless. But the fact that you cannot do anything to solve the problem does not mean there is nothing you can do.

The physician hears from the nurses how depressed John is. He waits for a quiet moment to enter his room. "I'm dying," John says. The silence is hard to bear. "Don't fool me doctor, I know it, I feel it." "Yes John, you're dying," the doctor says. No news is broken. They both know. Silence again. The doctor does not avoid John's eyes. "Are you afraid?" "No, not afraid, I'm so angry. I'm too young to die. My wife and children, they need me. I cannot die." "Whom can you talk with?" "Nobody, my wife always tries to cheer me up. She does not want to hear. Everybody is telling me to stay positive. I'm sick of it." Finally John has the chance to talk about his experience without being told what to do and what to feel. There is not much to respond, but to provide a space for expression. After a while he stops talking. "Thank you doctor for listening," he says, "I needed that so much."

What to do when there is nothing that can be done: be present. The first element needed for presence is safety. One cannot share an experience unless there is enough safety. Confidentiality is only a part of that. In the middle of a busy ward one cannot share more than a reassuring smile. For a serious conversation the patient must know you have the time to listen. The depth of the conversation corresponds to the time frame provided.

A second element is space. Experience does not need a solution, it needs space. John needed a space in which he could share his feelings. What he did not need were all those people who tried to talk his feelings out of his head. Sometimes you hardly need words, as long there is a space in which experience can be expressed.

Time and space are not enough. Recognition is also needed. The patient has to feel that he is heard and acknowledged in his experience. In John's case the doctor asks if he is afraid, acknowledging his fear. It turns out that he is not afraid but angry. Clarifying someone's experience allows the feeling of being understood. The only criterion for understanding is that the patient feels understood.

1.1.5 Coping

In order to understand the patient's perspective it is important to know what strategies people have to deal with illness and the associated emotions. In psychological terms this is called "coping."

There are two domains of coping, corresponding to the axis of "information" and "experience." One is problem-oriented coping, the other emotion-oriented coping. Most important is to realize that people differ in their coping styles.

1.1.5.1 Problem-Oriented Coping

When the doctor tries to explain to Peter what is wrong, she notices he hardly listens. "I don't really want to know," Peter says. "You probably know what is best for me. Just tell me what to do."

Lisa comes to the doctor's office with a huge pile of papers, from the Internet. All night she has been searching for information about her disease. In Canada, she knows, they started an experimental therapy. "Can I have that here too?"

Some people want to know all about their disease, some prefer not to know. Both coping styles are to be accepted.

Louise has finished her third cycle of chemo-

therapy, with no results at all. The doctor informs her he is running out of therapeutic options. Louise insists. She wishes to fight to the very end. The doctor reluctantly admits, there is still a possibility for treatment, but there are many side effects and very little chance of benefit. "I want it,", Louise says, "I don't want to give up."

Maria comes on time for her appointment. For more than 2 months she has been suffering from severe pain, she reports. The doctor does not understand why she did not come earlier. "Well," she says, "we had this appointment, so I waited."

In coping with problems some people are very active, others are more passive. In most cases different coping strategies only need to be understood and accepted.

1.1.5.2 Emotion-Oriented Coping

In the case of a severe disease not all problems can be solved immediately and some problems are clearly beyond any solution, as in the case of the death of a loved one. Apart from coping with the problem, we also need to cope with the emotion (see Fig. 2).

People have basically two strategies to deal with emotions, either to distract their attention away from it or to attend to the emotion. Both can be done alone or together with others. Examples of distraction are doing something pleasant, chattering, reading a book or listening to music. Some of these strategies can be problematic. The other way to deal with emotion is attending to it, giving it a space to heal. Examples are crying, talking with someone who listens, walking by the sea or in the woods, or keeping a diary.

None of these strategies is superior to the other. It is with the degree of liberty to move through the four quadrants of the diagram that one can be more comfortable with uncomfortable feelings. The first task of the caregiver is to respect the preferred coping styles of the patient. Only then he can invite the patient to broaden his repertoire and to try other coping strategies.

1.2 Conclusions

Where communication gets stuck and irritation and frustration arises, the communication compass may be of help. Are we stuck because of the different perspectives between clinicians and patient? Are we stuck because of a confusion between information and experience? Are we unable to listen to a patient's experience or have we lost our perspective? When communicational difficulties arise, one has to pause; if one has been lost, a compass can help.

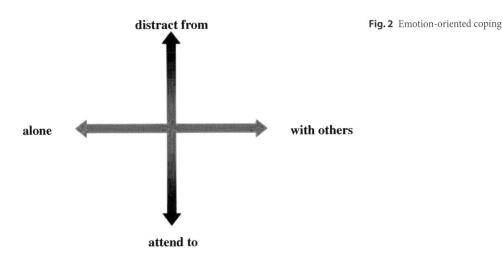

Fig. 2 Emotion-oriented coping

2 Motivating for Cancer Prevention

J. Cornuz, R. Bize

Recent Results in Cancer Research, Vol. 168
© Springer-Verlag Berlin Heidelberg 2006

Summary

Effective habit change usually requires a combination of psycho-educational, behavioural, and social learning strategies. Motivational interview and shared decision making are likely to be the most efficient approaches. Assessing the current motivation can be based on the transtheoretical model of change (TTM) with the goal to move from one behaviour to another healthier one. In a daily busy clinical practice, brief counselling interventions of one to three visits can substantially help patients change problematic behaviours, particularly in the areas of smoking cessation and exercise. The acronym FRAMES has been used to define the elements of an effective brief intervention which helps to trigger the patient motivation to change; giving Feedback based on a thorough assessment; helping the patient take Responsibility for changing; giving clear Advice on what behaviour must change; offering a Menu of options for making the change; expressing Empathy for the ambivalence and difficulty in making changes; enhancing Self-efficacy to foster commitment and confidence. This chapter reviews relevant aspects of clinician–patient communication with regard to cancer prevention, especially smoking cessation and exercise.

2.1 Introduction

This chapter focuses on the possibilities and limits of consultations addressing cancer prevention and discusses how persons can be motivated to change unhealthy behaviour. We outline the syntheses, recommendations and conclusions from landmark studies and reviews [1–4] on the integration of counselling techniques in clinical practice and discuss two major problematic behaviours, i.e. smoking and sedentary lifestyle.

The scientific literature provides data suggesting that promotion of effective clinical interventions is possible [2–4]. A meta-analysis of controlled trials of patients without diagnosed diseases showed that counselling helps patients to make behavioural changes [1]. The percentage of improvement of study participants in an experimental compared with a control group was 44% for smoking or alcohol cessation, 38% for nutrition or weight control, and 42% for other behaviours. In this review, interventions are divided into three categories: (1) adding a behaviour, such as nutritional supplement (e.g. calcium, folic acid or vitamin E), exercise and increasing physical activity, breast self-examination; (2) eliminating non-addictive behaviour, such as fats and excessive calories in the diet; (3) eliminating addictive behaviour, such as smoking and excessive alcohol use. The multivariate analysis showed that the best impact was produced by using behavioural techniques, particularly tailored interventions, rewarding for self-monitoring, and using several communication channels, such as media combined with personal communication [1].

Strategies to motivate for cancer prevention can be divided into three broad categories of patient education and counselling: psycho-educational; behavioural; and social learning [3,4].

2.1.1 Psycho-educational Counselling

As pointed out by experts, patient counselling and education focuses on transmitting factual information and advice [3,4]. Psycho-educational counselling goes beyond the simple exchange of facts to also include discussion of patients' emotions, values, and attitudes. Below, we outline three conceptual models that are represented in psycho-educational patient education and counselling [4].

2.1.1.1 Health Belief Model

Clinicians will be most effective if they understand their own cultural beliefs and the beliefs of their patients [3,4]. A single message is unlikely to be effective for all patients, meaning that the message must be delivered in a specific cultural context.

Accordingly, it is important for clinicians to explore the health beliefs that patients have formed through their personal experiences and attitudes toward health-related issues. In many instances, the health beliefs of patients may differ considerably from those of the clinician, and in these situations, a sub-optimal counselling exchange is likely to occur and compliance with recommendations is less likely [3,4].

2.1.1.2 Motivational Interviewing

"Motivation" is the probability that a person will enter into, continue, and adhere to a specific change strategy [5]. The fundamental concept underlying motivational interviewing is that patients are not all the same in their level of motivation for change. Furthermore, motivation for change is not considered to be a fixed personality trait, but rather a dynamic state that can change over time.

Motivational interviewing therefore incorporates an initial stage of assessing each individual's unique readiness for change, followed by subsequent tailored counselling that addresses that person's motivation with the ultimate objective being to assist them in positive behaviour change. This approach is particularly important in those who are either ambivalent or reluctant to change [4,5].

2.1.1.3 Shared Decision Making

The shared decision making model begins from the premise that an informed patient is better able to participate in decision making for their health [3,4]. Tools that facilitate the implementation of this counselling approach include interactive video tapes or computer programs that educate patients on key facts relating to complex medical decisions.

These types of instruments often include patients describing their perspective on health issues and have been demonstrated to be well received by patients in formal evaluation [6].

2.1.2 Behavioural Counselling

The fundamental concept underlying behavioural counselling is that certain behaviours are triggered by events or cues encountered in daily life [3,4,7]. Recognizing this, the likelihood of modifying behaviour through counselling that ignores such determinants is low.

The behavioural counselling intervention actively involves the patient in a process of personal reflection and learning to identify the cues that trigger behaviours [8]. The provision of information by the clinician to the patient is often insufficient; instead, behavioural counselling encourages the patient to undertake a process of self-assessment and discovery using instruments such as daily logs and self-administered questionnaires that attempt to uncover the cues underlying behaviours. The clinician can then review this material with the patients to help them develop a plan for either modifying the triggering factors, or modifying their reaction to the trigger. The clinician and patient can also work together to identify ways of modifying both the rewards and the adverse consequences associated with adopting new behaviours and abandoning old ones [9].

2.1.3 Social Learning

Social pressure can be an effective motivator for change [10]. The social support derived from belonging to a group of individuals who are seeking similar behaviour modification is a powerful means for change.

The help of peers, mentors or support groups, and the shared exchange of information, experiences, and personal strategies are central elements of the social learning model [3,4,10].

2.1.4 Using a Combination of Strategies

While each of preceding counselling approaches have merit, it is likely that a combination of strategies should be used in most cases [3,4,11]. Indeed, a study of physical activity counselling demonstrated that a combined approach was superior to a simple information strategy [12].

2.1.5 Brief Counselling Interventions

Brief counselling interventions can often lead to positive changes and have been proven to be effective in certain areas, such as smoking, exercise and hazardous alcohol use [3–5]. Below, we provide the FRAMES mnemonic that summarizes the elements of a brief intervention helping to trigger the patient motivation to change [4,5,13].

- Giving Feedback based on a thorough assessment
- Helping the patient take Responsibility for changing
- Giving clear Advice on what behaviour must change
- Offering a Menu of options for making the change
- Expressing Empathy for the ambivalence and difficulty in making changes
- Evoking Self-efficacy to foster commitment and confidence

The following sections present these interventions and support the clinician in identifying and assisting patients who are ready to accept a change.

2.2 How to Motivate Smokers to Quit

Smoking is associated with a range of diseases, causing a high level of morbidity and mortality. It represents one of the leading causes of preventable death with more than 3 million smokers worldwide dying each year from smoking-related illnesses. Stopping smoking has major health benefits. Smokers who quit before the age of 35 can expect a life expectancy only slightly less than those who have never smoked. Quitting at any age provides both short- and long-term benefits, with those who do so in middle age gaining improvements in health and reducing their excess risk of death. Despite the well-known health consequences of tobacco and the benefits of quitting, a quarter to a third of the adults in industrialized countries continue to smoke [14]. Although a majority of current smokers wish to quit smoking and effective interventions exist [15], very few request or receive formal smoking cessation interventions. Physicians are in a unique position to intervene; yet studies suggest that smokers are not consistently identified or treated in clinic settings [16]. In the following sections we overview interventions with smokers presenting in a primary care setting. This overview draws heavily from recent clinical practice guidelines for treating tobacco use and dependence, which were based on a qualitative and quantitative review of published clinical research [16–18].

2.2.1 General Recommendations

Even brief advice to quit offered by a physician produces abstinence rates of up to 5%–10%, which would have a significant public health impact if it were provided routinely [19, 20]. Unfortunately, surveys of smokers indicate that less then 50% receive such advice from their physicians [16, 19]. One reason why physicians hesitate to advise smoking cessation is that they be-

Table 1 The "5 A's" for smoking cessation intervention (from [15])

Ask about tobacco use	Identify and document tobacco use status for every patient at every visit
Advise to quit	In a clear, strong and personalized manner urge every tobacco user to quit
Assess willingness to make a quit attempt	Is the tobacco user willing to make a quit attempt at this time?
Assist in quit attempt	For the patient willing to make a quit attempt, use counselling and pharmacotherapy to help him or her quit
Arrange follow-up	Schedule follow-up contact, preferably within the first week after the quit date

come demoralized because they see that only few of their patients follow their advice. Although this is an understandable reaction due to an unrewarded behaviour, physicians should realize that even when their advice does not produce an immediate quit attempt by a patient, it may very well move the patient further towards the decision to quit smoking. Smoking cessation should be considered as a process of change through successive stages requiring counselling tailored to smokers' motivation to quit. Application of this model improves physicians' performance and the effect on 1-year smoking cessation [21].

Each smoker should therefore be encouraged to completely abstain from smoking and should be warned that other tobacco products, such as smokeless tobacco, are associated with significant health risks. Recently, smoking reduction has also been proposed as an alternative approach for smokers [22]. Even though such an approach seems promising, especially for heavy smokers who suffer from tobacco-related diseases such as chronic obstructive pulmonary disease, its effectiveness has still to be demonstrated. Before getting such evidence, the recommended clinical attitude should be to advise smokers to quit. Indeed, it is unlikely that a once-heavy smoker would be able to maintain light or infrequent

smoking without resorting to his or her old smoking patterns. Even lighter smoking (fewer than five cigarettes per day) has been associated with elevated health risks [23]. Strategies aimed at gradual reduction of smoking, versus quitting "cold turkey", appear to lead to continued craving and prolonged withdrawal symptoms in tobacco users; and smokers compensate by taking more and/or deeper puffs per cigarette when they attempt to reduce their smoking.

Clinical practice guidelines recommend that physicians follow the "5 A's" (see Table 1) in initiating assessment and intervention with tobacco users [15].

Every patient should be asked about his/her smoking status during each visit/consultation. As the guidelines stipulate, the physician then advises the patient to quit smoking with a clear ("It is important for you to quit smoking now, and I can help you. Cutting down while you are ill is not enough.") and strong statement ("As your physician, I need you to know that quitting smoking is the most important thing you can do to protect your health now and in the future. The clinic staff and I will help you."). The advice should also be personalized for the patient, highlighting his/her particular situation. For example, the advice may be tied to the patient's health ("Your smoking is not only prolonging your cough, it is putting you also at risk for long-term respiratory problems, such as chronic bronchitis or emphysema.") or the impact smoking might have on children ("You are putting your children at risk of asthma, ear infections and other diseases by exposing them to second-hand smoke.").

2.2.2 Intervention for Smokers Unwilling to Quit

Intervention efforts will not be successful without sufficient motivation or "readiness" to quit smoking on the part of the smoker. For the patient who is presently unwilling to quit smoking, recommending entering a smoking cessation programme may be premature and ineffective. The US practice guidelines suggest following the "5 R's" motivational intervention as listed in Table 2 [15]. The "5 R's" for enhancing motiva-

Table 2 Recommendations to enhance motivation to quit tobacco—the "5 R's" (from [15])

Relevance	Encourage the patient to indicate why quitting is personally relevant, being as specific as possible. Motivational information has the greatest impact if it is relevant to a patient's disease status or risk, family or social situation (e.g. having children in the home), health concerns, age, gender, and other important patient characteristics (e.g. prior quitting experience, personal barriers to cessation).
Risks	The clinician should ask the patient to identify potential negative consequences of tobacco use. The clinician may suggest and highlight those that seem most relevant to the patient. The clinician should emphasize that smoking low-tar/low-nicotine cigarettes or use of other forms of tobacco (e.g. smokeless tobacco, cigars, and pipes) will not eliminate these risks. Examples of risks are:
	Acute risks: Shortness of breath, exacerbation of asthma, harm to pregnancy, impotence, infertility, increased serum carbon monoxide.
	Long-term risks: Heart attacks and strokes, lung and other cancers (larynx, oral cavity, pharynx, oesophagus, pancreas, bladder, cervix), chronic obstructive pulmonary diseases (chronic bronchitis and emphysema), long-term disability and need for extended care.
	Environmental risks: Increased risk of lung cancer and heart disease in spouses; higher rates of smoking by children of smokers; increased risk for low birth weight, SIDS, and respiratory infections in children of smokers.
Rewards	The clinician should ask the patient to identify potential benefits of stopping tobacco use. The clinician may suggest and highlight those that seem most relevant to the patient. Examples of rewards follow:
	Improved health; food will taste better; improved sense of smell; save money; feel better about yourself; home, car, clothing, breath will smell better; can stop worrying about quitting; set a good example for children.
Roadblocks	The clinician should ask the patient to identify barriers or impediments to quitting and note elements of treatment (problem solving, pharmacotherapy) that could address barriers. Typical barriers might include:
	Withdrawal symptoms; fear of failure; weight gain; lack of support; depression; lack of enjoyment
Repetition	The motivational intervention should be repeated every time an unmotivated patient visits the clinic setting. Tobacco users who have failed in previous attempts should be told that most people make repeated quit attempts before they are successful.

tion to quit smoking comprise relevance, risks, rewards, roadblocks, and repetition.

2.2.3 Preparation for Quitting

The physician who has the opportunity to assist the patient's quit attempt, should include in the intervention the following elements (Table 3):
1. Helping the patient with a quit plan
2. Providing practical counselling (problem solving/skills training)
3. Providing intra-treatment social support
4. Helping the patient to obtain extra-treatment social support
5. Recommending the use of approved pharmacotherapy
6. Providing supplementary materials

The physician should then provide the patient with some basic didactic information about quitting smoking. (1) Smoking represents an addiction to nicotine. Therefore smoking cessation must be undertaken as seriously as one would approach any other drug addiction. Willpower alone is insufficient. The patient must make quitting smoking his/her top priority. (2) The goal should be total tobacco abstinence after the quit date. (3) The patient can expect to experience unpleasant nicotine withdrawal symptoms (e.g. mood disturbance, insomnia, irritability,

Table 3 Recommendations during preparation for quitting to smoke ("STAR" acronym [15])

1. Set a quit date as soon as possible

2. Tell family, friends, and co-workers about quitting and request understanding and support

3. Anticipate challenges to the planned quit attempt (including nicotine withdrawal symptoms), particularly during the critical first few weeks

4. Remove tobacco products from his/her environment and, prior to quitting, avoid smoking in places where spending a lot of time (e.g. work, home, car)

difficulty concentrating, increased appetite and weight gain). For most individuals, these symptoms peak within a few days of quitting and dissipate within 1 or 2 weeks. (4) The physician can help the patient identify "high-risk" or dangerous situations. These are events, internal states, or activities that increase the risk of smoking or relapse due to their past association with smoking (e.g. negative emotional states, being around other smokers, drinking alcohol). These situations should be avoided early on, if possible. (5) The physician can help the patient select cognitive and behavioural coping skills to use when experiencing an urge (or "craving") for cigarettes. Examples of cognitive coping skills are: reminding him/herself reasons for quitting; telling him/herself that urge will pass; and repeating the phrase, "Smoking is not an option." Behavioural coping skills include: leaving the situation, engaging in some distracting activity, taking deep breaths, and seeking social support.

The physician should also provide support within the clinic by: (1) encouraging the patient in the quit attempt (e.g. remind the patient that effective tobacco dependence treatments are now available; underline that one-half of all people who have ever smoked have now quit; communicate belief in the patient's ability to quit); (2) communicating caring and concern (e.g. ask how the patient feels about quitting; directly express concern and willingness to help; be open to the patient's expression of fears of quitting, difficulties experienced, and ambivalent feelings); (3) encouraging the patient to talk about the quitting process by asking the patient's reasons for quitting, concerns or worries about quitting,

success the patient has achieved, and difficulties encountered while quitting.

Eventually, the patient should be assisted with obtaining social support outside of the clinic environment. The clinician should train the patient in solicitation skills (e.g. practice requesting social support from family, friends, and co-workers; help for a patient in establishing a smoke-free home) and prompt support seeking (e.g. help the patient identify supportive others, inform patients of community resources such as hotlines). A busy physician may be tempted to hand one or more of the available self-help booklets to a smoker, instead of providing the personal advice called for by the "5 A's". However, clinical practice guidelines found that there was insufficient evidence for the effectiveness of the use of self-help materials alone [15].

2.3 How to Motivate Sedentary People to Be More Active

A sedentary lifestyle increases the risk of developing many diseases [24–27], particularly colon cancer and breast cancer. A sedentary lifestyle has become more and more prevalent during the last decade, as shown for example by successive "Swiss Health Surveys" [28]. In 2002, up to two-third of Swiss people reported that they practiced less physical activity than is minimally recommended [29, 30] (30 minutes per day of moderate intensity physical activity, such as brisk walking, or 3×20 minutes per week of vigorous intensity physical activity, such as jogging or other forms of cardio-respiratory training). It has been estimated that a sedentary lifestyle is annually responsible for 1.4 million disease cases, 2,000 deaths and 1.6 billion Swiss francs of treatment costs [31].

The efficacy of primary care physicians in changing unhealthy lifestyle habits has already been demonstrated in other fields (smoking cessation for example), particularly when they have been adequately trained [21]. With regard to physical activity promotion in a primary care setting, more than 20 original papers [32–51] and ten reviews of the literature have been published [52–61]. There is a fair amount of evidence

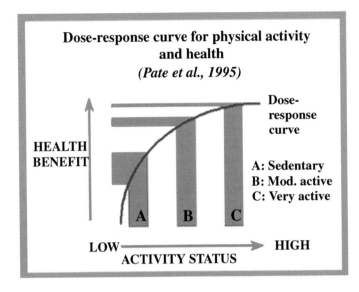

Fig. 2.1 Dose-response curve for physical activity and health, (Adapted from Pate et al. 1995

that multi-session interventions are efficient, at least in the short term. As demonstrated by Eakin et al. in a recent review [62], little is known, on the other hand, about physicians' compliance to physical activity counselling. However, many health agencies (The Department of Health and Human Services, Centres for Disease Control and Prevention, American Academy of Family Physicians, The American Heart Association) do recommend that physicians provide their sedentary patients with counselling about the health benefits of regular physical activity.

2.3.1 General Recommendations

Since many health benefits occur even with a small increase in physical activity among previously sedentary people (Fig. 1), effort should concentrate on broadly promoting everyday life activities.

Lack of time is the main barrier for primary care physicians to deliver counselling. We therefore suggest a differentiated approach according to their degree of achievable involvement.

The first strategy is broad-based, with a systematic screening for sedentary lifestyles, for example in the waiting room, conceived for phy-

sicians who have the opportunity to integrate physical activity promotion as a priority topic in their practice.

Sedentary patients who are unmotivated to change their physical activity behaviour should then benefit from a brief consciousness-arousing session and be invited to read related information. Those who are motivated should benefit from a structured counselling session, receive written information, and a physical activity prescription using the existing structures within their environment (walking groups, fitness centres etc.).

The second strategy is more case-oriented and allows limited time resources to be focused on sedentary patients who suffer from conditions known to be improved by physical activity (e.g. obesity). As for the first strategy, interventions should then be tailored to patients' motivation becoming more active.

Physicians' follow-up is probably a key determinant of efficacy and should be widely encouraged. Follow-up can be based on successive "physical activity diaries", which describe every physical activity lasting more then 10 min during a week, or on more objective data, according to patient's preference, e.g. measures by means of a pedometer. Such instruments, however, should not discourage patients because of too

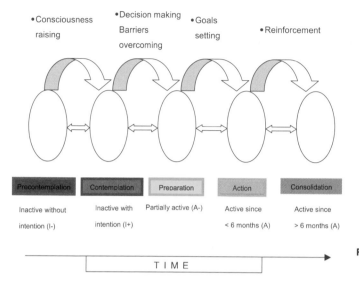

Fig. 2.2 Different stages of change

high expectations and should not substitute the patient's self-perceptions of physical activity levels.

2.3.2 How to Proceed

2.3.2.1 Assessing the Patient's Current Physical Activity

During the interview, the physician explores the patient's daily life in terms of physical activity practice, for example, by asking his/her patient to describe the progress of a usual weekday or a weekend. The physician identifies opportunities of the patient to move by his own physical means. This approach should help the patient to recognize by himself his sedentary lifestyle, and provide at the same time ideas on how to integrate, step by step, more physical activity in his daily life.

Setting an objective does not always mean reaching the minimal international standard recommendations. More important is to tailor an achievable goal, which is adapted to the previous experiences and present motivation of the patient.

A more systematic but less personalized way to assess the current level of physical activity of a patient is the use of internationally standardized questionnaires, such as the IPAQ (www.ipaq. ki.se). Patients, prior to an appointment during which this theme will be tackled, could, for example, fill in such a questionnaire in the waiting room or at home.

2.3.2.2 Assessing the Current Motivation— Transtheoretical Model of Change

According to the transtheoretical model of change (TTM) of Prochaska and di Clemente, moving from one behaviour to another healthier one is a complex process. The different stages of this model are called the stages of change, and are described in Fig. 2.

The stage at the lower end of motivation is called the precontemplation stage, where the person is not physically active and does not intend to become more active. Next is the contemplation stage, where the person is not physically active but considers becoming more active soon. The third stage is the preparation stage, where the person is physically active but does not meet the criteria of international recommendations for frequency, duration or intensity of physical activity. The fourth is the action stage, where the person meets the criteria for being considered

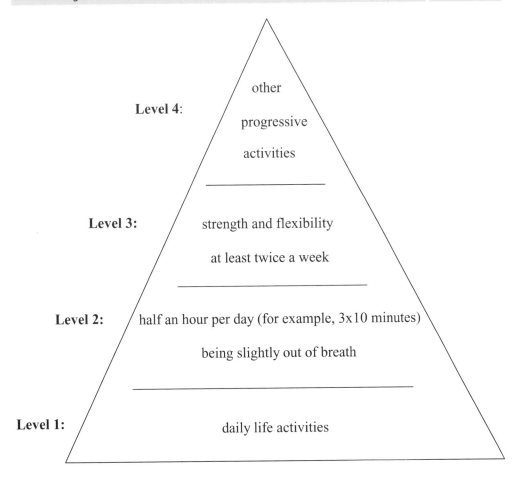

Fig. 2.3 Recommendations based on the four-level pyramid model

as sufficiently physically active, but only for less than 6 months. The last stage is the consolidation stage, where the person is physically active enough, for more than 6 months. Relapses also belong to this process.

Progression through these stages depends on three key elements:

1. The person must recognize his/her own goals in this process of change.
2. The person has to favour the pros against cons of adopting the new behaviour.
3. The person must be confident enough to reach the goal, despite anticipated barriers.

People are often subjected to fluctuating levels of motivation during the whole process. The role of the physician is to reinforce motivation through counselling, in accordance with the level of motivation.

Precontemplation Here, physicians have to raise consciousness about health benefits of a regular physical activity of moderate intensity. They also have to explore the potential barriers to this behaviour change and advise the patient on how to overcome them.

Contemplation Physicians should describe the different ways of becoming more physically active. Recommendations are based on a four-level pyramid model, similar to the one used for nutritional recommendations (Fig. 3).

Priorities must, however, be understood in a flexible manner in accordance with the clinical situation. Sometimes strength and coordination training may be more relevant than cardio-respiratory fitness, for example, when fall prevention is the main objective. People who are not yet retired may sometimes omit the first level, because they are already active (even if they do not meet the recommendations) in their daily working life. Physical activity counselling calls for a differentiated approach by the physician, who knows the medical, psychosocial, and structural context of his patients; risk management of physical activity belongs to this evaluation. A medical examination is moreover recommended independently from the health status for men above 45 years and women above 55 years who engage in a new vigorous cardio-respiratory training.

2.3.3 Techniques for a More In-Depth Counselling: How to Manage Ambivalence

In this section, we provide a list of the most frequent arguments against becoming more physically active and ways to counteract them in a non-oppositional manner.

"I feel very well despite/thanks to my sedentary lifestyle."
Diseases that are favoured by inactivity develop insidiously, without health or well-being being impaired at the beginning. Regular physical activity reduces the risk of diseases and it improves well-being and body perception.

"I don't have enough time to exercise and I prefer doing something else during my leisure time."
Physical activities of moderate intensity, such as bicycling or walking, are already beneficial to health. There are many opportunities to practice them without taking too much time (getting out of the bus sooner, park one's car 10 minutes away from the workplace, climbing stairs rather than taking the elevator, etc.). Physical activity can also be integrated into other leisure activities (museum visit, city touring, etc.).

"I feel a lack of energy and I don't feel like beginning a physical activity."
Movement and sport stimulate the whole body. When practiced at an adequate intensity, they can become a source of well-being and the reluctance to practice them is quickly surmounted.

"I will never be a good sportsman/woman and I don't dare to begin with it."
A health-enhancing physical activity is not a competition. You only have to be regular in order to improve your well-being. The body adapts quickly to new solicitations. To improve your health, it is important to practice physical activities with which you feel comfortable.

"Sport does not entertain me."
Do not practice sport, but movement, which can be associated with numerous other activities. When practiced with a group, they favour social contacts. Cultural visits also offer an opportunity to walk. Walking around does not take too much time and allows appreciating the environment. It is recommended to diversify your activities, because tediousness may produce withdrawal.

"The risk of injury and disease frequency increase with sport."
Physical activity-related risks are low. They only rarely have serious consequences and accidents are often due to a lack of common sense (poor preparation, inadequate equipment, imprudence, haste). The choice of the activity, the moderation of its intensity, and preparation largely reduce the risk of accident.

"Sport is too demanding."
Inactive people sometimes find the first physical activities quite demanding. A slow increase in intensity and duration of exercise prevents exhaustion and allows the body to adapt. Then, after each new physical activity, the tiredness disappears faster and faster and the practice of these movements becomes easier and more pleasant.

"Sport is too expensive."
Physical activity and sport can be free. Everyday life activities, for example, do not require specific equipment.

"A healthy diet is all that I need to stay well."

A healthy diet is beneficial for health. But it only provides the body with combustibles (energy) that feed the power station, the muscles. The combination of well-balanced physical activity and diet is the better insurance for well-being and health.

"Physically active people live longer and then increase health costs."

On the contrary, physically active people remain autonomous, have fewer accidents, consult physicians and are hospitalized less frequently and for shorter periods. They consequently induce less health system costs.

"I don't have any opportunity to exercise in the neighbourhood."

Physical activity does not necessitate a specific infrastructure. You only have to combine it with your everyday life activities (way to work, shopping, visit exhibitions or friends).

"Sport is very dangerous."

The risk of dying suddenly during sport is very low for moderate-intensity physical activities. Ninety-five percent of myocardial infarctions are not preceded by increased physical activity.

2.3.4   Risk Management in Physical Activity Promotion

Physical activity-related risks are low and largely lower than the health benefit of regular moderate-intensity physical activity. For example, for sport, it is important that someone who wishes to increase their training is well informed and counselled, that he structures his progress and that he adequately organizes his contests and training sessions in order to avoid any overloading. More than 90% of myocardial infarction events did not follow a physical activity; however, the risk may increase for a while immediately after exercising, although this risk concerns almost exclusively non-trained people. This underlines the preventive role of being regularly active. Every healthy person can have a daily physical activity of moderate intensity without visiting a physician first.

In this case, the potential risk can be evaluated through the Physical Activity Readiness Questionnaire (PAR-Q, see the end of this section).

Someone who answered once or many times "yes" to these questions can exercise, but she should be advised to visit a physician beforehand. The general practitioner will then evaluate more precisely the risk profile of the person, and will be able to advise her to undertake appropriate physical activities.

A medical visit is also recommended to men above 45 years and women above 55 years who would like to start new intense physical activities.

When indicated, the medical visit should be based on the following elements:

1. Thorough cardiovascular history taking
2. Thorough physical examination
3. Resting ECG
4. Level of blood pressure
5. Cholesterol (>35 years)

The patient should be sent to a specialist for complementary examinations in case of a positive cardiovascular history, of cardiac or vascular murmurs, of rhythm disturbance signs in the history, or of an abnormal resting ECG.

2.3.5   Physical Activity Readiness Questionnaire

For most people, physical activity should not pose any problem or hazard. PAR-Q has been designed to identify the small number of adults for whom physical activity might be inappropriate or those who should get medical advice concerning the type of activity most suitable for them (Table 4).

2.4   Conclusion

Smoking and a sedentary lifestyle represent two of the leading causes of preventable cancers. Stopping smoking and practising regularly physical activity have major short- and long-term health benefits. Despite these well-known health conse-

Table 4 Physical Activity Readiness Questionaire

Common sense is your best guide in answering these questions. Please read them and check the yes/no opposite the question if it applies to you		
Has your doctor ever said you have heart trouble?	YES	NO
Do you frequently have pains in your heart and chest?	YES	NO
Do you often feel faint or have spells of severe dizziness?	YES	NO
Has a doctor ever said your blood pressure was too high?	YES	NO
Has your doctor ever told you that you have a bone or joint problem such as arthritis that has been aggravated by exercise, or might be made worse with exercise?	YES	NO
Is there a good physical reason not mentioned here why you should not follow an activity program even if you wanted to?	YES	NO
Are you over age 65 and not accustomed to vigorous exercise?	YES	NO
If you answered YES to one or more questions...	If you have not recently done so, consult with your physician by telephone or in person before increasing your physical activity and/or taking a fitness test.	
If you answered NO to all questions...	If you answered PAR-Q accurately, you have reasonable assurance of your suitability for exercising.	

quences and the fact that effective interventions exist for motivating patients to change their unhealthy behaviours [15], very few individuals request or receive formal preventive interventions. Physicians are in a unique position to intervene. Since the scientific literature provides enough evidence to promote effective clinical interventions, physicians should address this crucial issue in their daily clinical practice.

References

1. Mullen PD, Simons-Morton DG, Ramirez G et al. (1997) A meta-analysis of trials evaluating patient education and counseling for three groups of preventive health behaviors. Patient Educ Couns 32:157
2. Becker MH (1985) Patient adherence to prescribed therapies. Med Care 155:1877
3. Lang RS, Hensrud DD (eds) (2004) Clinical preventive medicine, 2nd ed. AMA Press, Chicago, IL
4. Duffy DF (1999) Techniques to incorporate counselling into the medical encounter. In: Rose BD (ed) UpToDate. UpToDate, Waltham, MA
5. Miller WR, Rollnick S (1991) Motivational interviewing: preparing people to change addictive behavior. The Guilford Press, New York
6. Barry MJ, Fowler FJ, Mulley AG et al. (1995) Patient reaction to a program designed to facilitate patient participating in treatment decisions for benign prostatic hyperplasia. Med Care 33:771
7. DiMatteo MR (1991) The psychology of health, illness and medical care: an individual perspective. In: Brooks, Cole (eds) Pacific Grove
8. Gordon GH, Duffy FD (1998) Educating and enlisting patients. J Clin Outcomes Manage 5:45–50
9. Russell ML (1986) Behavioral counseling in medicine: strategies for modifying at-risk behavior. Oxford University Press, New York

10. Bandura A (1986) Social foundations of thought and action: a social cognitive theory. Prentice Hall, Englewood Cliffs

11. Waitzkin H (1985) Information giving in medical care. J Health Soc Behav 26:81–101

12. Marcus BH, Goldstein MG, Jette A et al. (1997) Training physicians to conduct physical activity counseling. Prev Med 26:382–388

13. Miller WR, Rollnick S (2002) Motivational interviewing: preparing people for change. Guilfort Press, New York

14. www.who.int/tobacco/resources/publications/tobacco_atlas/en

15. Fiore MC, Bailey WC, Cohen SJ, Dorfman SF, Goldstein MG, Gritz ER et al (2000) Treating tobacco use and dependence. Clinical Practice Guideline. US Department of Health and Human Services, Public Health Service, Rockville, MD

16. Thorndike AN, Rigotti NA, Stafford RS, Singer DE (1998) National patterns in the treatment of smokers by physicians. JAMA 279:604–608

17. Raw M, McNeill A, West R (1998) Smoking cessation guidelines for health professionals. Thorax 53 [Suppl]:S1–S19

18. Rigotti N (2002) Treatment of tobacco use and dependence. N Engl J Med 346:506–512

19. US Department of Health and Human Services (2000) Reducing Tobacco Use: A Report of the Surgeon General.US Department of Health and Human Services, Centers for Disease Control and Prevention, National Center for Chronic Disease Prevention and Health Promotion, Office on Smoking and Health, Atlanta, GA

20. Lancaster T, Stead L, Silagy C et al. (2000) Effectiveness of interventions to help people Stop smoking: findings form the Cochrane Library. BMJ;321:355–358

21. Cornuz J, Humair JP, Seematter L, Stoianov R, van Melle G, Stalder H et al (2002) Efficacy of resident training in smoking cessation: a randomized, controlled trial of a program based on application of behavioral theory and practice with standardized patients. Ann Intern Med 136:429–437

22. Kunze M (2000) Maximizing help for dissonant smokers. Addiction 95 Suppl 1:S13–7

23. Rosengren A, Wilhelmsen L, Wedel H (1992) Coronary heart-disease, cancer, and mortality in male middle-aged light smokers. J Intern Med 231:357–362

24. US Department of Health and Human Services (1996) Physical Activity and Health: A Report of the Surgeon General. US Department of Health and Human Services, Centers for Disease Control and Prevention, National Center for Chronic Disease Prevention and Health Promotion, Atlanta, GA

25. Hoidrup S, Sorensen TI, Stroger U, Lauritzen JB, Schroll M, Gronbaek M (2001) Leisure-time physical activity levels and changes in relation to risk of hip fracture in men and women. Am J Epidemiol 154:60–68

26. JR, Jr., Jackson AW, Bazzarre TL, Milne D, Blair SN (1999) A one-year follow-up to physical activity and health. A report of the Surgeon General. Am J Prev Med 17:24–30

27. P, Borms J Health enhancing physical activity (Perspectives—The multidisciplinary series of physical education and sport Science, vol 6). Meyer & Meyer Sport, Oxford

28. Martin BW, Mäder U, Calmonte R (1999) Représentation, connaissances et attitude de la population suisse concernant l'activité physique: Résultats de l'enquête sur l'exercice physique 1999. Schweiz Z Sport-med Sporttraumatol 47:165–169

29. RR, Pratt M, Blair SN, Haskell WL, Macera CA, Bouchard C et al. (1995) Physical activity and public health. A recommendation from the Centers for Disease Control and Prevention and the American College of Sports Medicine JAMA 273:402–407

30. Martin BW, Lamprecht M, Calmonte R, Raeber PA, Marti B (2000) Taux d'activité physique de la population suisse: niveaux et effets sur l'état de santé. Prise de position scientifique rédigée en commun et publiée par les partenaires suivants: Office fédéral du sport (OFSPO), Office fédéral de la santé publique (OFSP), Office fédéral de la statistique (OFS), Réseau santé et activité physique Suisse. Schweiz Z Sport-med Sporttraumatol 48:161–162

31. Martin BW, Beeler I, Szucs T, Smala AM, Brügger O, Casparis C et al. (2001) Répercussions économiques du rapport entre santé et activité physique: premières estimations pour la Suisse. Schweiz Z Sport-med Sporttraumatol 49:87–89

32. Jimmy G, Martin BW (2005) Implementation and effectiveness of a primary care based physical activity counselling scheme. Patient Educ Couns 56:323–331

33. DN, Lazaro CM, Meier RV (1989) The feasibility of behavioral risk reduction in primary medical care. Am J Prev Med 5:249–256

34. KJ, Long BJ, Sallis JF, Wooten WJ, Pratt M, Patrick K (1996) A controlled trial of physician counseling to promote the adoption of physical activity. Prev Med 25:225–233

35. LC, Paglia MJ, German PS, Shapiro S, Damiano AM (1995) The effect among older persons of a general preventive visit on three health behaviors: smoking, excessive alcohol drinking, and sedentary lifestyle. The Medicare Preventive Services Research Team. Prev Med 24:492–497

36. BS, Lynch WD (1993) The effect of physician advice on exercise behavior. Prev Med 22:110–121

37. (1994) Effectiveness of health checks conducted by nurses in primary care: results of the OXCHECK study after one year. Imperial Cancer Research Fund OXCHECK Study Group. BMJ 308:308–312

38. Swinburn BA, Walter LG, Arroll B, Tilyard MW, Russell DG (1998) The green prescription study: a randomized controlled trial of written exercise advice provided by general practitioners. Am J Public Health 88:288–291

39. AC, Ochera JJ, Hilton SR, Bland JM, Harris T, Jones DR et al. (1996) Prevention in practice: results of a 2-year follow-up of routine health promotion interventions in general practice. Fam Pract 13:357–362

40. MG, Pinto BM, Marcus BH, Lynn H, Jette AM, Rakowski W et al. (1999) Physician-based physical activity counseling for middle-aged and older adults: a randomized trial. Ann Behav Med 21:40–47

41. FC, Jamrozik K (1998) Advice on exercise from a family physician can help sedentary patients to become active. Am J Prev Med 15:85–94

42. W, Hillsdon M, Thorogood M, McArdle D (1998) Cost-effectiveness of a primary care based physical activity intervention in 45–74 year old men and women: a randomised controlled trial. Br J Sports Med 32:236–241

43. BH, Goldstein MG, Jette A, Simkin-Silverman L, Pinto BM, Milan F et al. (1997) Training physicians to conduct physical activity counseling. Prev Med 26:382–388

44. JP, Williams SJ, Drew JA, Wright BL, Boulan TE (1995) Longitudinal effects of preventive services on health behaviors among an elderly cohort. Am J Prev Med 11:354–359

45. Graham-Clarke P, Oldenburg B (1994) The effectiveness of a general practice-based physical activity intervention on patient physical activity status. Behavior Change 11:132–144

46. Kelly RB 1(988) Controlled trial of a time-efficient method of health promotion. Am J Prev Med 4:200–207

47. EL, Morgan RW (1979) Exercise prescription: a clinical trial. Am J Public Health 69:591–595

48. SJ (1993) Educational and behavioral strategies related to knowledge of and participation in an exercise program after cardiac positron emission tomography. Patient Educ Couns 22:47–57

49. M, Thorogood M, White I, Foster C (2002) Advising people to take more exercise is ineffective: a randomized controlled trial of physical activity promotion in primary care. Int J Epidemiol 31:808–815

50. CR, Kerse N, Arroll B, Robinson E (2003) Effectiveness of counselling patients on physical activity in general practice: cluster randomised controlled trial. BMJ 326:793

51. Writing Group for the Activity Counseling Trial Research Group (2001) Effects of physical activity counseling in primary care: the Activity Counseling Trial: a randomized controlled trial. JAMA 286:677–687

52. EG, Glasgow RE, Riley KM (2000) Review of primary care-based physical activity intervention studies: effectiveness and implications for practice and future research. J Fam Pract 49:158–168

53. CB, Menard LM (1998) A systematic review of physical activity promotion in primary care office settings. Br J Sports Med 32:11–16

54. M, Thorogood M (1996) A systematic review of physical activity promotion strategies. Br J Sports Med 30:84–89

55. Simons-Morton DG, Calfas KJ, Oldenburg B, Burton NW (1998) Effects of interventions in health care settings on physical activity or cardiorespiratory fitness. Am J Prev Med 15:413–430

56. Ashenden R, Silagy C, Weller D (1997) A systematic review of the effectiveness of promoting lifestyle change in general practice. Fam Pract 14:160–176

57. Eden KB, Orleans CT, Mulrow CD, Pender NJ, Teutsch SM (2002) Does counseling by clinicians improve physical activity? A summary of the evidence for the US Preventive Services Task Force. Ann Intern Med 137:208–215

58. DA, Hanratty B (2001) The effect of physical activity advice given in routine primary care consultations: a systematic review. J Public Health Med 23:219–226

59. Petrella RJ, Lattanzio CN (2002) Does counseling help patients get active? Systematic review of the literature. Can Fam Physician 48:72–80

60. Riddoch C, Puig-Ribera A, Cooper A (1998) Effectiveness of physical activity promotion schemes in primary care: a review. Health Education Authority, London

61. Smith BJ, Merom D, Harris P, Bauman A (2002) Do primary care interventions to promote physical activity work? The National Institute of Clinical Studies, Melbourne

62. Eakin EG, Smith BJ, Baumann AE (2005) Evaluating the population health impact of physical activity interventions in primary care—Are we asking the right questions? J Phys Act Health 2:197–215

3 Communication in Genetic Counselling for Breast/Ovarian Cancer

S. Dolbeault, C. Flahault, D. Stoppa-Lyonnet, A. Brédart

Recent Results in Cancer Research, Vol. 168
© Springer-Verlag Berlin Heidelberg 2006

Summary

Cancer genetic counselling represents a very special situation of interaction between the geneticist and the counselee, marked by a number of specificities that account for its complexity. Cancer genetic counselling has multiple repercussions, such as identification of a deleterious genetic mutation associated with a high probability of developing breast and/or ovarian cancer, the implementation of preventive measures ranging from close surveillance to the decision to perform mutilating prophylactic surgical procedures, or the impact of the information on the other members of the counselee's family also concerned by the genetic risk. This chapter is based on a review of the literature that has been rapidly growing over recent years and on our clinical expertise as psycho-oncologists and geneticists. We will first present the reasons that make the information so critical. These reasons are both objective (complexity of the genetic information per se, difficulties of understanding the concept of risk) and subjective (information given to people with an emotionally charged family history and a perception of risks closely linked to their representation of cancer). At the same time, the counsellees are charged with the transmission of this information to members of their own family. We will then discuss the various modalities of communication in this setting. While unidirectional transfer of information from the geneticist to the counselee has been the preferred method in cancer genetics for a long time, a model based on patient-centered communication is more adequate in predictive medicine and allows shared decision making. In all cases, the different professionals involved in the process have to learn how to work in a performing cohesion. We also present the main guidelines on the subject and the various underlying objectives with regard to information delivery and the subject's personal experience. Although the psychological impact of genetic counselling consultations raises a number of questions, the results of preliminary studies are reassuring, demonstrating psychological benefits. However, a number of aspects concerning communication in predictive medicine remain to be investigated and improved.

3.1 Introduction

The discovery of the BRCA1 cancer-susceptibility gene in 1994 (Miki et al. 1994) and BRCA2 in 1995 (Wooster et al. 1995) now allows identification of individuals with a cancer predisposition mutation by performing DNA mutation analysis. There has always been a popular belief concerning hereditary transmission of breast cancer, which has been supported by this scientific progress and mediatization of this breakthrough has led to an increased awareness of the concept of family risk, resulting in a growing demand for genetic counselling and genetic testing (Bottorff et al. 1998; Holloway et al. 2004).

However, known inherited gene mutations are only involved in 5% of cancer cases (King et al. 1993). Presymptomatic genetic testing is therefore not appropriate for the majority of women with a family history of breast cancer. The indication for gene mutation testing first has to be discussed in preliminary genetic counselling consultation.

Breast cancer genetic testing was initially proposed in the context of research protocols. In this setting, sustained follow-up of the counselees not only helped them to anticipate the outcome of the genetic test, but also allowed interventions in the case of psychological distress. Meanwhile, breast cancer genetic testing has become available in routine clinical practice, despite the fact that it is not yet clear how to adequately inform patients about their personal breast cancer risk and the pros and cons of genetic testing (Green et al. 2004). Moreover, the long-term impact of genetic counselling on psychological well-being and health behaviour is still largely unknown.

In this chapter, we will discuss the psychological aspects of cancer genetic counselling and review the current knowledge concerning its psychological impact. We will try to define the optimal modalities of communication between geneticist and counselee, and demonstrate that the subject's understanding of a risk can be modified by individual psychological characteristics, which must therefore be taken into account.

3.2   Complexity of Cancer Genetic Counselling

Genetic counselling is a highly complex process due to both objective and subjective factors. The information provided in the context of cancer genetic counselling, including the concept of risk, is objectively complex. More subjectively, this information must be provided to an individual, mostly a woman, who is often emotionally affected by a family history of cancer and who will have to consider the pros and cons of the necessities of surveillance or preventive surgical options. In addition, the counsellee also has to act as a messenger to the members of the family, whose relationships might subsequently be modified by the information.

3.2.1   Objective Factors

3.2.1.1   Complexity of the Information

The primary goal of genetic counselling is to inform individuals about cancer risk and cancer prevention in order to reduce morbidity and mortality (Pieterse et al. 2005). More specifically, genetic counselling should enhance their knowledge and encourage favourable health behaviours, i.e. by adequate objective risk perception with a level of anxiety that does not impair understanding or appropriate medical surveillance.

The information provided in cancer genetic counselling is complex for different reasons. First, the counselee is faced with a very large quantity of information. The various national guidelines for cancer genetic predisposition management (see in Bortoff et al. 1998; Richards et al. 1995; Eisinger et al. 2004) represent a considerable amount of information that must be presented to and understood by the counselee. After the genetic counselling visit, the subject should know: (1) the purpose of the test; (2) the risk of the test (e.g. consecutive insurance problems); (3) the uncertainty of the test; (4) the risk that the test may reveal an unexpected finding; and (5) the consequences of a positive test (e.g. impact on family members) (Butow et al. 2004). Therefore, one can expect that the counselee is often overwhelmed by such a body of information and that psychosocial aspects are neglected in the consultation.

The information is also based on a very abstract and unusual medical terminology; it is in fact difficult to translate molecular genetic findings into lay terms and the general population has a poor understanding of Mendelian genetics. Another element of complexity is the rapidly growing scientific progress and the still existent methodological limitations and lack of long-term follow-up of current methods (Eisinger et al. 2004). Finally, the information concerning the consequences of genetic testing is also complex. Genetic testing for breast/ovarian cancer susceptibility offers a potential benefit of early detection of cancer, reduction of uncertainties, and relief if the test provides negative results. However, genetic testing also entails potential risks, such as the risk of failure of preventive interventions, adverse psychological reactions, social and occupational discrimination or inappropriate health surveillance behaviour (Brédart et al. 1998). When discussing these aspects, the genetic counselling consultation should allow individuals to make informed medical decisions about whether or not to be tested and the adoption of appropriate preventive strategies.

3.2.1.2 Concept of "Risk"

The information provided in a cancer genetic counselling consultation essentially concerns risks. The concept of risk is traditionally defined as "the probability of (occurrence of) a negatively valued event" (Julian-Reynier et al. 2003). In the context of cancer genetics, information about risk is particularly complex, as cancer risk information concerns multiple risks (e.g. all epidemiological and personal risk factors, risk of the predisposing gene running in the family or of inheriting a genetic mutation, risks associated with the prognosis of cancer and preventive/early detection interventions), and most risk estimators are associated with uncertainty. For example, if a person in a cancer family is found not to carry the predisposing gene, the probability of developing a sporadic cancer (i.e. not linked to a hereditary component) remains equivalent to that of individuals in the general population. Risk estimators also comprise uncertainty, particularly for penetrance of genes. Estimates of penetrance values of BRCA genes appear to vary between 60% and 85% at age 70 for breast cancer and between 10% and 40% for ovarian cancer (Struewing et al. 1997; Ford et al. 1998; Antoniou et al. 2003).

Certain non-contributive or unexpected results can lead to a highly paradoxical situation, because the subject expects a result which should decrease uncertainty about her genetic status, but the results sometimes increase uncertainty by information she does not know how to use. A good example is the discovery of variants of uncertain clinical significance (VUCS). VUCS refers to alterations of genetic sequences whose

risk consequences are often unknown (they differ from inconclusive results in that inconclusive results mean that no BRCA1/2 mutation is detected) (van Dijk et al. 2004b).

3.2.2 Subjective Factors

Cancer genetic risk information must be integrated by individuals who are often emotionally affected by a family history of cancer, life experiences and psychological characteristics which determine the understanding of the information and the perception of the risk.

3.2.2.1 Impact of Prior Experiences and Emotions

The experience of a family history of cancer is frequently associated with feelings such as fear, low self-esteem, anger, guilt, grief, and embarrassment. This experience must be taken into account as a possible barrier in the education about cancer genetic risk.

On the one hand, studies of women with a high risk for breast cancer due to a family history of the disease in first-degree relatives have found that these women experienced high levels of worry about their risk (Lerman and Schwartz 1993; Audrain et al. 1997). Levels of anxiety about cancer, on the other hand, have been shown to be associated with inaccurate perception of breast cancer risk in women at risk (Hopwood 2000).

While the emotional impact of a family experience of cancer is variable, it is likely to generate a certain amount of distress during counselling (van Dijk et al. 2004a).

3.2.2.2 Perception of Risk

Prior to genetic risk counselling, only a minority of women have an accurate perception of their risk of developing breast cancer, and the majority either overestimate or underestimate their risk (Hopwood 2000). Cross-cultural differences have been demonstrated, with a much greater risk overestimation in the USA than in the UK.

Risk overestimation is also high in Latin countries (Huiart et al. 2002; Gil et al. 2003).

Cognitive biases, individual preconceptions (and misconceptions), life experiences, cultural context, the subject's general outlook (e.g. pessimism, locus of control), as well as social biases, such as family history and related beliefs of being vulnerable, may also influence the interpretation of risk information (Bottorff et al. 1998).

Providing up-to-date and accurate risk estimates to the counselee is one of the main goals of genetic counselling; but how is cancer risk perceived after counselling?

Studies evaluating risk perception vary widely in their definition of risk accuracy leading to inconsistent results (Hopwood et al. 2003b; van Dijk et al. 2004a). In a 1-year prospective study of 158 women aged 18–45 years with a confirmed lifetime risk of breast cancer of 1 in 6 or greater, the proportion of women with accurate personal risk perceptions based on "gambling" odds (1 chance in x) significantly improved after risk counselling (Hopwood et al. 2003b). "Gambling" odds was the method of reporting perceived risk with the best level of risk accuracy and women preferred this format. However, the concept of lifetime risk was understood by only 44% of counselees.

Using open-ended, semi-structured face-to-face interviews, van Dijk and coworkers (2004a) showed that the level of risk perception accuracy depended on the leniency of the criterion applied, being either an exact match with the verbal label or more global high versus low level of risk estimation.

In a prospective study performed on 108 women receiving genetic counselling, women's risk perceptions after counselling were significantly lower than pre-counselling, but still significantly higher than the actual risk information communicated (Gurmankin et al. 2005).

Kelly and coworkers (2004) examined changes in perceived breast cancer risk from post-counselling (1–2 days after counselling) to post-result (1 week after receipt of test results), and found that the perceived risk decreased in those tested negative, but remained unchanged in those tested positive. They concluded that individuals may assume that they have a hereditary mutation until they receive contrary test results; this may be interpreted as a coping method of assuming the worst in order to manage anxiety or as defensive pessimism.

In conclusion, van Dijk and coworkers (2004a) emphasized that the level of perceived risk accuracy might be a limited outcome for assessing the effectiveness of genetic counselling and that it would be preferable to identify which emotions, cognitions, and behavioural intentions are elicited by the risk information and whether they are congruent with the goals of counselling (i.e. adopting medically appropriate behaviours, reporting a moderate level of distress after counselling).

3.2.2.3 Messenger Role

A further difficulty involves communication of cancer genetic information within the family. The counselee becomes a messenger of sensitive information to other family members. However, little is known about this process (Tercyak et al. 2001, 2002; Blandy et al. 2003).

While cancer genetic counselling is addressed to an individual, it also concerns the whole family. At first sight, the person who consults may appear to be the person primarily concerned, but the implications obviously surpass the individual case. As already discussed, the subject expects a result from the visit (answers to questions about the cause of the disease, reduction of the anxiety related to uncertainty, information concerning prevention, etc.), but there are no genetics without family and the information therefore inevitably concerns the person's descendents, ascendants, as well as other members of her own generation.

This observation raises the very complex question concerning ownership of the information: does this information belong exclusively to the one who consults or does it immediately belong to the whole family? Is the person aware of this twofold ownership and/or has the rest of the family already questioned a possible genetic predisposition?

These ethical issues have a number of consequences on the practical organization of cancer genetic counselling and must be investigated before performing the test, especially before providing the results. A thorough investigation of the personal motivations, as well as perception of the implications for the rest of her family, has therefore to be an integral part of genetic counselling.

3.3 Communication in Cancer Genetic Counselling

The three main objectives of doctor–patient communication in medicine are: the creation of a trustful interpersonal relationship, exchange of information, and treatment-related decisions (Ong et al. 1995). The primary objective of cancer genetic counselling is exchange of information. However, to obtain an adequate level of informed consent, to minimize distress, improve satisfaction, and promote appropriate preventive behaviour, other aspects must also be taken into account, especially an evaluation of the patient's understanding of the information provided and of the emotional reactions induced by this information.

3.3.1 Communication Models

Various communication models have been described in general medicine. In cancer genetic counselling, the "rational" model now appears to be predominant. This model emphasizes the importance of the information derived from the medical profession, which must enable the counselee to take an informed decision. This model only partly satisfies the expectations of counselees. As Pieterse and coworkers (2005) stressed, the major issues for counselees were to discuss their own and/or their family members' risk of cancer, to receive information about early detection of cancer and preventive actions, and to determine the risk for their children, or of transmitting an increased susceptibility to their children. Other important expectations included the need for emotional support, to reduce anxiety, to obtain help in discussing genetic risk issues in the family and to receive information about the counselling and testing procedure. The "rational" model therefore appears to be fairly limited.

Borttoff and coworkers (1998) described a model of "shared medical decision-making", which advocates a partnered decision-making in which the professional engages with the client to achieve an understanding of the meaning of the genetic risk, by taking into account the individual's expectations and representations, and to reach a medical decision considering the various available medical solutions and their consequences.

In the particular setting of cancer genetic risk communication, probability and contextual approaches have been proposed. The probability approach provides numerical information in the form of a numerical risk, such as absolute risk (assessing a discrete estimate of risk), relative risks (assessing risk in comparison to another individual or group), odds ratio or ratios (frequency of events, proportions, percentages, probabilities) and verbal descriptions of risk magnitude (unlikely, higher risk than average, higher risk than another woman in the population). Visual displays, such as line graphs, pie charts and bar graphs reveal data patterns and may also communicate uncertainty. A preference for quantitative information has been highlighted and a combination of visual displays and numerical and written information improves the perceived usefulness of the information and the perception accuracy (Julian-Reynier et al. 2003). The contextual approach communicates risk with reference to the patient's medical history and the consequences of the health problem, providing, for example, information about the causes of the disease and the severity of its consequences, or using testimonies or videos.

3.3.2 Communication Guidelines

Various guidelines for risk counselling are now available (Richards et al. 1995; Eisinger et al. 2004). A multistep process has been proposed (Julian-Reynier et al. 2003), starting with assessment of the counselee's preconceptions, knowledge, preferences, expectations, anxiety and coping style in order to tailor the risk communication process. The information to be given to the counselee (risk, magnitude, uncertainty, format) is then selected and ordered so that it can be put in perspective with other disease risks, using several formats. Lastly, feedback from the consultation is provided by means of standardized tools that complement the consultation (leaflet, videos, CD-ROM), and a personal letter summarizing the consultation.

Bottorff and coworkers (1998) also highlighted strategies such as relationship and trust building, history taking, explanation of risk, and risk assessment. Efforts are made to help counselees understand the meaning of risk estimates in relation to other life events, and to emphasize that the risk of developing the disease is not the same as the risk of dying from the disease.

We underline the considerable role, both technical and emotional, played by the clinical geneticist and genetic counsellor (Lobb et al. 2004), as well as their multiple tasks. They routinely initiate contact with the family, obtain a pedigree, obtain consent from living relatives to access medical records, confirm relevant medical data, ascertain family beliefs about the inheritance pattern, advise family members of these risks and options and arrange clinical screening (Richards 1993). From a subjective point of view, counselees are confronted with the difficulty of providing complex medical information while dealing with the emotional repercussions of belonging to a family with a cancer history and learning about one's own risk status and its consequences. Management of all of these dimensions, even in a 1h consultation, is a challenge.

3.3.3 Organization of Cancer Genetic Counselling in France

Various models of cancer genetic counselling, depending on national or regional expertise and resources, have been developed (Hopwood 2005).

In France, for example, the various professionals working in the field of cancer genetics, forming the "Genetics and cancer" group, have proposed guidelines for cancer genetic counselling, based on a multidisciplinary organization in which the various healthcare professionals meet with the counselee at various times.

The first meeting is a long consultation, for which the counselee is encouraged to attend with a certain amount of preparation (maximum of information about the family history of cancer). The counselee is invited to attend the visit with one or several members of the family. The counselee's family tree is constructed and a maximum of information is obtained about all cancers in the family; then, the geneticist describes the objectives of genetic counselling, the existence of genes and their possible alteration, the concept of risk, the implications of genetic testing, the various expected results and their consequences, the concept of specific surveillance and possible prophylactic surgical procedures aimed to decrease the risk of developing cancer. Finally, the geneticist provides information about the risk of the family members and advice concerning the transmission of this information. At the end of the visit, the geneticist provides the counselee with a fairly precise estimate of the probability that she carries the BRCA1 or BRCA2 genetic alteration. The counselee is given an information brochure, summarizing the information provided orally, which can be read at home and shared with other members of the family.

Usually, it is proposed not to take the blood sample for genetic testing immediately, as the counselee is given a period of reflection of about 2 months during which she is encouraged to attend a visit with a member of the psycho-oncology team. The psycho-oncology interview is an opportunity for the counselee to review her motivation to undergo genetic testing, to explain her expectations and to investigate the subject's representations of cancer, especially in the light of her family history, and to share her level of information and her integration of the information presented at the first meeting with the geneticist. The psycho-oncology interview investigates the counselee's perception of risk, her capacity to anticipate the results of genetic testing, her desire to transmit the information received to her family, and, more globally, the model of family communication. It also assesses the psychological impact of the genetic risk and the possible risk of psychiatric disturbance related to this situation. The interview sometimes leads to the decision not to perform the genetic test or at least to postpone it.

The second meeting with the geneticist, often shorter than the first, confirms the counselee's motivation and reinforces the main information. After understanding how the counselee and her family experience this period of reflection, the geneticist answers any of the patient's remaining questions. A letter summarizing the genetic information provided during the consultation is then handed to the counselee; this can be especially helpful for the counselee to recall this information and to transmit it to the family.

The psycho-oncologist may follow the counselee during this period, but is usually only consulted at the time of delivery of the genetic test results.

In every case, geneticists and psycho-oncologists meet regularly to pool their information in order to achieve a global understanding of the counselee's expectations, values, and choices and the possible psychological difficulties. Written summaries are included in the counselee's file, allowing sharing of information collected by the various professionals involved.

It should be underlined that the geneticist not only informs on the genetic situation but also takes part in the organization of the next steps of the process. After presenting the different possibilities to reduce the counselee's risks, surveillance or preventive surgery, he participates in the practical organization of the medical exams or further consultations with members of the multidisciplinary medical team.

This cancer genetic counselling model is continually evolving, especially in view of the recent arrival, in France, of newly trained genetic counsellors, which will modify the distribution of roles between the various professionals involved.

3.3.4 Impact of Organization on Outcomes

Although cancer genetic counselling services vary in terms of staffing and/or organization, evidence suggests that the context of risk counselling has a less important impact on psychological outcomes than expected (Hopwood et al. 2003a). In terms of organization, a multidisciplinary team achieved a significantly greater improvement of risk knowledge than cancer genetic counselling

administered by a surgical department (Brain et al. 2003). The different models currently implemented should be further evaluated, looking for the most convenient one.

3.3.5 Process and Content of Familial Breast Cancer Genetic Consultations

Butow and Lobb (2004) conducted a major study, examining in detail the process and content of genetic counselling in initial consultations with women from high-risk breast cancer families. Over 158 consultations of women unaffected and affected with breast cancer, conducted in 10 familial breast cancer clinics throughout Australia, were audiotaped and transcribed. A detailed coding system was developed to cover all facts thought to be important to be elicited from or conveyed to the consultant, and all behaviours thought to facilitate active involvement and expression of emotional concerns.

This analysis evidenced that the average genetic counselling session was 61 min [comparable to that of European clinics (Hopwood et al. 2003a)], that patients spoke on average one-third of the session and consultants demonstrated consistently good practice in providing detailed information on essential aspects related to familial breast cancer. The authors noted that, although the woman's agenda was frequently elicited, other subjects were tackled less frequently, namely the women's decision to discuss the results with other family members or emotional concerns such as those relating to prior experiences of loss and grief. Considering the predominant role played by information processing in cancer genetic counselling, it has to be stressed that passive listening reduces understanding and interactivity should therefore be stimulated. Moreover, training in or self-monitoring of behaviours known to facilitate understanding (checking women's medical knowledge, checking understanding, explaining medical terms, inviting questions, summarizing, and using diagrams) may assist clinical geneticists and genetic counsellors to further develop these skills.

3.4 Consequences of Cancer Genetic Counselling

3.4.1 Psychological Impact

Major questions still remain unanswered: What is the psychological impact of genetic counselling? Does cancer genetic counselling induce psychological morbidity? What is known about the short-term and longer-term impact?

In a systematic review (Butow et al. 2003), genetic counselling and testing appeared to produce psychological benefits. Carriers of mutations in cancer predisposition genes did not experience any significant increase of depression and anxiety after disclosure of their mutation status, while non-carriers experienced significant relief. If general distress levels for counselees are comparable with community samples, cancer-specific worries are increased in women at risk compared with those without a family history (Hopwood, 2005). On the other hand, women who were tested, but who refused to be informed about the results, seemed to be at greater risk of poorer psychological outcome (Lerman et al. 1998).

3.4.2 Satisfaction with Cancer Genetic Counselling

Assessing the satisfaction of 36 counselees with cancer genetic counselling in The Netherlands, Bleiker and coworkers (1997) found generally high levels of satisfaction with the different aspects assessed. The areas identified as needing further attention were related to the information regarding the possible impact of genetic counselling and testing on daily life, communication between the clinical geneticist and other healthcare workers, and psychosocial support during and after genetic counselling.

3.4.3 Psychological Consequences in Relation to Communication Style

Two factors appear to be particularly important when communicating risk information: the individual's affective response to risk information and the communicator's skill and sensitivity in disclosing the results (Borttoff et al. 1998).

3.4.3.1 The Individual's Affective Response to Risk Information

Greater attention should be paid to ways of coping with test results at the very first contact with the genetic counselling service. Younger women, those without a history of cancer, and those who are first in their family to apply for genetic counselling for breast/ovarian cancer, have been shown to withdraw prematurely from cancer genetic counselling (Bleiker et al. 2005). They do not appear to have elevated levels of distress, but they seem to have doubts about their (in)ability to cope with a possible unfavourable test outcome.

3.4.3.2 Communication Skills in Disclosing Genetic Test Results

Various skills should be considered when communicating cancer genetic information or test results, such as the counsellor's sensitivity to individual and cultural differences, the language used (avoiding medical jargon), the ability to provide emotional support, and the counsellor's own anxiety level, which has been found to be inversely correlated with the counselee's capacity for understanding (Lobb et al. 2001).

Further research is needed to examine the counsellor's communication style in relation to the psychosocial impact of cancer genetic counselling (Hopwood 2005). The few available studies are presented below.

In a multicentre study, Lobb and coworkers (2005) showed that clinical geneticists and genetic counsellors achieved a certain degree of standardization in communicating information, but showed a diversity of skills, i.e. communication behaviours that facilitate understanding, active involvement, partnership building, and addressing emotional concerns. These variations in counselling style resulted in differences of patient's depression, 4 weeks after the counselling session. However, there was no association between the way genetic risk was communicated and women's accuracy of risk recall or satisfaction with the consultation.

Butow and coworkers (2004) highlighted that increased use of supportive and counselling communications increased anxiety about cancer, suggesting that emotional issues may be raised without adequate resolution. It may be helpful for consultants to be able not only to assess psychological stress, but also to keep checking how the woman is coping during the consultation and to provide adequate support.

3.4.4 Communication in the Family

The effect of risk communication is also reflected in subsequent disclosure of risk information in the family (Hopwood 2005). There is a need to improve knowledge about communication strategies within the family and their impact on family relationships and family members' reactions. Very few studies have been conducted in this field.

Tercyak and coworkers (2001) evaluated the psychological impact of the parental communication of the result of BRCA1/2 testing. Mothers (versus fathers) and subjects with the highest levels of general emotional distress more easily informed their children about the test results. Coping strategies after the test (both active and avoidant) were positively correlated with the post-counselling distress level. However, communication of the result to the children did not modify the counselee's level of distress, but increased their children's level of distress.

The same authors also evaluated the parent–child relationship and its impact on the communication of test results to the children (Tercyak et al. 2002). Older children appeared to be more frequently informed about the test results, and the communication style within the family seemed to predict the way mothers shared the information with their children (the test result was more frequently shared when the communication style between parents and children was more open), and was not modified by revelation of the result.

Blandy and coworkers (2003) showed that results of BRCA tests were generally adequately transmitted to the family; difficulties of transmission, however, correlated with a poorer understanding and a higher level of anxiety and avoidance. First-degree relatives were most frequently informed about the test results, but they only rarely requested genetic testing, which was essentially requested by sisters and daughters. The quality of family support and the level of understanding of the risk of transmission were positively and significantly correlated with the decision to perform the test in first-degree relatives.

In France, the bioethical legislation has recently considered this medical situation in which information elicited in one individual of a family concerns all its members. The latest bioethical law sets that the biomedical agency takes the responsibility to confer this information to the different family members: the transmission should proceed from doctor to doctor, and from them to family members (Public Health Policy, Biomedicine Agency, 2004).

3.5 Improvement of Cancer Genetic Counselling

Studies indicate that cancer genetic consultants present generally good practice in terms of the information they provide; however, they less frequently demonstrate attention or skills to deal with the subjective aspects of the genetic counselling, i.e. verifying the counselee's understanding of the information, assessing emotional reactions or attitudes of informed family members.

Biesecker and Peters (2001) proposed a working definition for genetic counselling consultations that defines the goals as "promoting understanding, achieving informed consent, facilitating decision-making, reducing psychological distress, restoring feelings of personal control and advancing adaptation to stress-inducing events".

These objectives are much more exhaustive than those regarding patient information. However, this definition raises new questions: What is the exact role of the geneticist or genetic counsellor, especially concerning the evaluation of emotional reactions or the provision of psychosocial support?

There is a growing number of guidelines for communicating risk, suggesting the need to develop and evaluate innovative communication strategies (Bottorff et al. 1998; Hopwood 2005). Genetic counsellors should also be encouraged to explore idiosyncratic risk beliefs, personal theories of inheritance, and personal or social support that underpin coping. Integration of risk information may be enhanced when emotional issues are addressed. Geneticists or genetic counsellors are confronted with the challenging task of providing objective information which is adapted to the individual, taking into account the individual's concerns and preferences. Counselees often express a marked need to receive more attention and information with regard to the possible impact of cancer genetic risk on their daily life and the availability of psychosocial support (Bleiker et al. 1997). These aspects do not seem to be sufficiently addressed in genetic consultations. Several key elements can improve communication.

3.5.1 Develop Aids to Recall and Transmit Information

We have stressed the double role of the information provided at the cancer genetic counselling visit, allowing the counselee to understand the risk for herself, before having to transmit the information acquired to her own family.

A growing number of field experiences and studies have reported the benefit of proposing on the spot or by means of documents (written documents or videos) a summary of the complex information presented during the visit. Hallowell and coworkers (1998) showed that counselees feel

a duty to share the information they obtain during genetic counselling to relatives, and warned about the risk of miscommunication (due to the counselee's difficulty to recall information). In a series of 400 interviews, 92% of subjects reported that the written summary facilitated their understanding and/or recall of the information.

Tools should be developed to alleviate the burden of information provision within the cancer genetic consultation; for example, information personally tailored to the individual's needs, characteristics and coping style (personalized letter, audiotape, computer-generated information, telephone services) or information/decision aids.

Even when the counselee is accompanied by other members of her family, she remains responsible for the information received and its transmission to the rest of the family. It is therefore important to develop ways of helping her to anticipate the information that he/she has to transmit, as well as in the transmission process itself.

Several modalities can be proposed, such as letters to families that can be sent by the doctor with the patient's consent, discussion with the patient during the visit about the content of the information to be transmitted and the way to transmit this information, or meetings with other members of the family to inform them during a consultation.

3.5.2 Improve Communication Style

One motivation for attending genetic counselling is to receive reassurance. Unaffected women cited information as reassuring, whereas affected women perceived the skills of the geneticists in listening, appearing caring and relaxed, as providing an independent source of support. It may therefore be more important to actively reassure affected women.

This supposes relational capacities which are not only innate, but which can be acquired by specific training, the so-called communication skills training (CST), which are based on analysis of fictional clinical situations (with actors simulating patients or as role plays between healthcare professionals) or real clinical situations which are audio-recorded and/or filmed and complemented by role play and supervisions (Balint groups or equivalent).

It is therefore important to increase the awareness of healthcare professionals, as early as possible, about CST or other ways of improving communication techniques.

3.5.3 Further Promote Multidisciplinary Collaboration

Various healthcare professionals are in contact with the counselee during the cancer genetic counselling process (geneticist, genetic counsellor, psycho-oncologist, etc.). Multidisciplinary meetings between healthcare professionals of these various fields enhance the understanding of the counselee: his/her values, motivations, capacity to integrate the information, personal perception of the risk, anticipation of the consequences of the test results, desire to transmit the information to other members of the family—all elements that contribute to the decision-making process.

3.5.4 Take Time

Although no data on these aspects are available, we can assume that the time devoted to assess the counselee's knowledge, perceived risk, information/emotional needs and preferred modalities of risk information is an important element of genetic risk counselling.

During a consultation, the geneticist or genetic counsellor should help counselees demystify genetics, and highlight how expertise in this field may answer many of their actual medical questions although some will remain unresolved and some will raise further issues still unaddressed. Such an approach may require time, which may be well invested, since it increases efficient information sharing.

3.6 Conclusions

There are insufficient data concerning optimal risk communication strategies. Recent research shows both consistency in information provision and deficiencies in specific communication skills. The need for personally tailored risk information seems a key element of successful genetic risk counselling (Hopwood 2005). Outcome studies on risk perception and psychological distress are insufficient to understand the complex communication and decision-making process in this context. Assessment of the risk counselling process is a new field and evaluation and comparison of various approaches therefore constitute a research priority. Outcome measures must also include decision-making and subsequent healthcare behaviours. In addition, communication within the family raises a number of difficulties that have not been sufficiently investigated yet.

There is a need to provide clear directions about how to ensure that the probabilistic nature of risk estimates is accurately transmitted and understood, and especially how the error-proneness of genetic tests is sensitively communicated (Bottorff et al. 1998).

References

1. Antoniou A, Pharoah PD, Narod S et al. (2003) Average risks of breast and ovarian cancer associated with BRCA1 or BRCA2 mutations detected in case Series unselected for family history: a combine analysis of 22 studies. Am J Hum Genet 72:1117–1130
2. Audrain J, Schwartz MD, Lerman C, Hughes C, Peshkin BN, Biesecker B (1997) Psychological distress in women seeking genetic counseling for breast-ovarian cancer risk: the contributions of personality and appraisal. Ann Behav Med 19:370–377
3. Biesecker BB, Peters KF (2001) Process studies in genetic counseling: peering into the black box. Am J Med Genet 106:191–198
4. Blandy C, Chabal F, Stoppa-Lyonnet D, Julian-Reynier C (2003) Testing participation in BRCA1/2-positive families: initiator role of index cases. Genet Test 7:225–233

5. Bleiker EM, Aaronson NK, Menko FH, Hahn DE, van Asperen CJ, Rutgers EJ, ten Kate LP, Leschot NJ (1997) Genetic counseling for hereditary cancer: a pilot study on experiences of patients and family members. Patient Educ Couns 32 :107–116

6. Bleiker E, Wigbout G, van Rens A, Verhoef S, van't Veer, Aaronson N (2005) Withdrawal from genetic counselling for cancer. Hereditary Cancer in Clinical Practice 3:19–27

7. Bottorff JL, Ratner PA, Johnson JL, Lovato CY, Joab SA (1998) Communicating cancer risk information: the challenges of uncertainty. Patient Educ Couns 33:67–81

8. Brain K, Norman P, Gray J, Rogers C, Mansel R, Harper P (2002) A randomized trial of specialist genetic assessment: psychological impact on women at different levels of familial breast cancer risk. Br J Cancer 86:233–238

9. Brédart A, Autier P, Audisio RA, Geragthy J (1998) Psycho-social aspects of breast cancer susceptibility testing: a literature review. Eur J Cancer Care 7:174–180

10. Butow PN, Lobb EA, Meiser B, Barratt A, Tucker KM (2003) Psychological outcomes and risk perception after genetic testing and counselling in breast cancer: a systematic review. Med J Aust 178:77–81

11. Butow PN, Lobb EA (2004) Analyzing the process and content of genetic counseling in familial breast cancer consultations. J Genet Couns 13:403–424

12. Public Health Policy (2004) Chapter 1: general principles Law reinforced n° 2004–800 of the 6th August 2004 related to bioethics. Biomedicine Agency

13. Eisinger F, Bressac B, Castaigne D, Cottu PH, Lansac J, Lefranc JP, Lesur A, Nogues C, Pierret J, Puy-Pernias S, Sobol H, Tardivon A, Tristant H, Villet R (2004) Identification and management of hereditary predisposition to cancer of the breast and the ovary (update 2004). Bull Cancer 91:219–237

14. Ford D, Easton DF, Stratton M, Narod S, Goldgar D, Devilee P, Bishop DT, Weber B, Lenoir G, Chang-Claude J, Sobol H, Teare MD, Struewing J, Arason A, Scherneck S, Peto J, Rebbeck TR, Tonin P, Neuhausen S, Barkardottir R, Eyfjord J, Lynch H, Ponder BA, Gayther SA, Zelada-Hedman M et al. (1998) Genetic heterogeneity and penetrance analysis of the BRCA1 and BRCA2 genes in breast cancer families The Breast Cancer Linkage Consortium. Am J Hum Genet 62:676–689

15. Gil F, Mendez I, Sirgo A, Llort G, Blanco I, Cortes-Funes H (2003) Perception of breast cancer risk and surveillance behaviours of women with family history of breast cancer: a brief report on a Spanish cohort. Psycho-Oncology 12: 821–827

16. Green MJ, Peterson SK, Baker MW, Harper GR, Friedman LC, Rubinstein WS, Mauger DT (2004) Effect of a computer-based decision aid on knowledge, perceptions, and intentions about genetic testing for breast cancer susceptibility: a randomized controlled trial. JAMA 292:442–452

17. Gurmankin AD, Domchek S, Stopfer J, Fels C, Armstrong K (2005) Patients' resistance to risk information in genetic counseling for BRCA1/2. Arch Intern Med 165:523–529

18. Hallowell N, Murton F (1998) The value of written summaries of genetic consultations. Patient Educ Couns 35:27–34

19. Holloway S, Porteous M, Cetnarskyj R, Anderson E, Rush R, Fry A, Gorman D, Steel M, Campbell H (2004) Patient satisfaction with two different models of cancer genetic services in south-east Scotland. Br J Cancer 90:582–589

20. Hopwood P (2000) Breast cancer risk perception: what do we know and understand? Breast Cancer Res 2:387–391

21. Hopwood P, van Asperen CJ, Borreani G, Bourret P, Decruyenaere M, Dishon S, Eisinger F, Evans DG, Evers-Kiebooms G, Gangeri L, Hagoel L, Legius E, Nippert I, Rennert G, Schlegelberger B, Sevilla C, Sobol H, Tibben A, Welkenhuysen M, Julian-Reynier C (2003a) Cancer genetics service provision: a comparison of seven European centres. Community Genet 6:192–205

22. Hopwood P, Howell A, Lalloo F, Evans G (2003b) Do women understand the odds? Risk perceptions and recall of risk information in women with a family history of breast cancer. Community Genet 6:214–223

23. Hopwood P (2005) Psychosocial aspects of risk communication and mutation testing in familial breast-ovarian cancer. Curr Opin Oncol 17:340–344

24. Huiart L, Eisinger F, Stoppa-Lyonnet D, Lasset C, Nogues C, Vennin P, Sobol H, Julian-Reynier C (2002) Effects of genetic consultation on perception of a family risk of breast/ovarian cancer and determinants of inaccurate perception after the consultation. J Clin Epidemiol 55:665–675

25. Julian-Reynier C, Welkenhuysen M, Hagoel L, Decruyenaere M, Hopwood P; CRISCOM Working Group (2003) Risk communication strategies: state of the art and effectiveness in the context of cancer genetic services. Eur J Hum Genet 11:725–736

26. Kelly K, Leventhal H, Andrykowski M, Toppmeyer D, Much J, Dermody J, Marvin M, Baran J, Schwalb M (2005) Using the common sense model to understand perceived cancer risk in individuals testing for BRCA1/2 mutations. Psycho-oncology 14:34–48

27. King MC, Rowell S, Love SM (1993) Inherited breast and ovarian cancer. What are the risks? What are the choices? JAMA 269(:1975–1980

28. Lerman C, Schwartz M (1993) Adherence and psychological adjustment among women at high risk for breast cancer. Breast Cancer Res Treat 28:145–155

29. Lerman C, Hughes C, Lemon SJ, Main D, Snyder C, Durham C, Narod S, Lynch HT (1998) What you don't know can hurt you: adverse psychologic effects in members of BRCA1-linked and BRCA2-linked families who decline genetic testing. J Clin Oncol 16:1650–1654

30. Lobb EA, Butow P, Barratt A, Meiser B, Tucker K (2005) Differences in individual approaches: communication in the familial breast cancer consultation and the effect on patient outcomes. J Genet Couns 14:43–53

31. Lobb EA, Butow PN, Barratt A, Meiser B, Gaff C, Young MA, Haan E, Suthers G, Gattas M, Tucker K (2004) Communication and information-giving in high-risk breast cancer consultations: influence on patient outcomes. Br J Cancer 90:321–327

32. Lobb EA, Butow PN, Meiser B, Barratt A, Gaff C, Young MA, Kirk J, Gattas M, Gleeson M, Tucker K (2003) Women's preferences and consultants' communication of risk in consultations about familial breast cancer: impact on patient outcomes. J Med Genet 40:e56

33. Lobb E, Butow P, Meiser B, Tucker K, Barratt A (2001) How do geneticists and genetic counsellors counsel women from high risk breast cancer families? J Genet Couns 10:185–199

34. Miki Y, Swensen J, Shattuck-Eidens D, Futreal PA, Harshman K, Tavtigian S, Liu Q, Cochran C, Bennett LM, Ding W, et al (1994) A strong candidate for the breast and ovarian cancer susceptibility gene BRCA1. Science 266:66–71

35. Ong LM, de Haes JC, Hoos AM, Lammes FB (1995) Doctor-patient communication: a review of the literature. Soc Sci Med 40:903–918

36. Pieterse A, van Dulmen S, Ausems M, Schoemaker A, Beemer F, Bensing J (2005) QUOTE-gene(ca): development of a counselee-centered instrument to measure needs and preferences in genetic counseling for hereditary cancer. Psycho-oncology 14:361–375

37. Richards MPM (1993) The new genetics: some issues for social scientists. Sociol Health 15:567–586

38. Richards MPM, Hallowell N, Green JM, Murton F, Statham H (1995) Counseling families with hereditary breast and ovarian cancer: a psychosocial perspective. J Genet Couns 4:219–233

39. Struewing JP, Hartge P, Wacholder S, Baker SM, Berlin M, McAdams M, Timmerman MM, Brody LC, Tucker MA (1997) The risk of cancer associated with specific mutations of BRCA1 and BRCA2 among Ashkenazi Jews. N Engl J Med 336:1401–1408

40. Tercyak KP, Peshkin BN, Streisand R, Lerman C (2001) Psychological issues among children of hereditary breast cancer gene (BRCA1/2) testing participants. Psycho-oncology 10:336–346

41. Tercyak KP, Peshkin BN, DeMarco TA, Brogan BM, Lerman C (2002) Parent-child factors and their effect on communicating BRCA1/2 test results to children. Patient Educ Couns 47:145–153

42. van Dijk S, Otten W, van Asperen CJ, Timmermans DR, Tibben A, Zoeteweij MW, Silberg S, Breuning MH, Kievit J (2004a) Feeling at risk: how women interpret their familial breast cancer risk. Am J Med Genet 131:42–49

43. van Dijk S, van Asperen CJ, Jacobi CE, Vink GR, Tibben A, Breuning MH, Otten W (2004b) Variants of uncertain clinical significance as a result of BRCA1/2 testing: impact of an ambiguous breast cancer risk message. Genet Test 8:235–239

44. Wooster R, Bignell G, Lancaster J, Swift S, Seal S, Mangion J, Collins N, Gregory S, Gumbs C, Micklem G (1995) Identification of the breast cancer susceptibility gene BRCA2. Nature 378:789–792

4

Informing About Diagnosis, Relapse and Progression of Disease – Communication with the Terminally Ill Cancer Patient

F. Stiefel, D. Razavi

Recent Results in Cancer Research, Vol. 168
© Springer-Verlag Berlin Heidelberg 2006

Summary

This chapter focuses on four crucial situations representing important challenges for physician–patient communication: diagnosis, relapse, progression of disease and terminal illness. The psychological aspects of each situation are discussed and a framework for communication is provided. The aim of the chapter is to invite the oncology clinician to think about these different stages of disease and to support him or her in the communication with the patient.

Communication with cancer patients is a difficult task in clinical practice and it is especially challenging when informing about diagnosis and prognosis, when relapse occurs or when the disease is progressing. Physician–patient communication has undergone considerable changes and has become—compared to decades before, when medicine was based on a more paternalistic model of care—a central duty and challenge of the oncology clinician. The following chapter aims to discuss key elements of communication in the above-mentioned specific situations; it is based on our clinical experience as psycho-oncologists and teachers of communication skills training (Razavi and Stiefel 1994; Stiefel and Razavi 1994; Razavi et al. 2003; Berney and Stiefel 2004; Delvaux et al. 2005; Voelter et al. 2005; Bragard et al. 2006).

4.1 Disclosing a Cancer Diagnosis

To face a diagnosis of malignant disease is an extreme stressor. What has been a silent and reliable body suddenly becomes a source of doubts and fears, disturbing—together with the associated investigations and therapeutic propositions—the psychological and social balance of man. However, reactions to these events vary considerably from individual to individual, depending on a variety of factors, such as personal resources, social support, coping and defence mechanisms, such as denial. In other words: individual strengths and vulnerabilities shape the response to the bad news of a cancer diagnosis. Communicating such a diagnosis, therefore, requires an adjustment to the individual information needs and coping capacities.

The oncologist often does not know the patient to whom a diagnosis of cancer has to be announced.. A few elements may therefore be of help for the evaluation of the patient's psychological state to which information will have to be adapted. The main question is, when communicating with a newly diagnosed cancer patient, whether he is a vulnerable patient to whom communication has to be especially tailored or whether he is a patient who may be informed in a standard way, taking into account the usual recommendations when announcing a cancer diagnosis (see next section).

Table 1 Indicators of psychological vulnerabilities of a patient

| Important patient's delay despite alarming physical symptoms |
| Inability to work or to assume other responsibilities |
| Occurrence of severe sleep or gastrointestinal disturbances |
| Experience of long-lasting periods of overwhelming emotions |
| Social withdrawal, substance abuse, self-destructive behaviour |

Table 2 Breaking bad news to the psychologically vulnerable patient

| Try to understand patient preferences with regard to information |
| Focus on the "essentials", use understandable words, avoid "jargon" |
| Provide a clear framework/management plan |
| Emphasize that beneficial therapeutic options exist |
| Invite patient to cope "day by day" and "step by step" |
| Inform about well-known medical experience with patient's disease |

4.1.1 Perceiving the Patient's Strengths and Vulnerabilities

As stated above, the oncologist may not know the patient for very long and it may be inadequate or impossible to obtain detailed biographical information before breaking bad news. A few elements, related to the current situation, may therefore be of help to quickly evaluate the psychological strengths and vulnerabilities of a patient (see Table 1).

The patient's delay between the occurrence of the first symptoms and consulting a physician is such an element. The longer the delay, the more likely the patient may have used denial; denial is directly related to psychological vulnerability. As a psychological defence mechanism, denial protects the individual from painful experiences he cannot bear (Weisman 1979). Other important elements concern the current state of the patient. Is he able to function in his professional and private life? Was he disturbed by the situation in a way that hampered his capacities to work or to care for the family? Was he able to maintain social contacts and activities or was he paralysed by the occurrence of the medical problems? Symptoms related to bodily functioning may also indicate a psychological vulnerability of the patient; how did she sleep and eat, did she suffer from gastro-intestinal symptoms, was she unable to relax? If patients are able to express their feelings, are the emotions in an adequate range or are they overwhelming the patient? If different elements indicate an important vulnerability, information should be carefully adapted to the individual.

4.1.2 Discussing Diagnosis with a Psychologically Vulnerable Patient

With a general clinical impression based on some of the above-mentioned elements and the verbal and non-verbal communication of the patient, the oncologist can identify the patient's strengths and vulnerabilities. If the clinician faces a vulnerable patient who seems to be very stressed and almost unable to cope, communication of the cancer diagnosis should be adapted in a way that the patient obtains the information he needs without increasing the psychological pressure (see Table 2). Communicating diagnosis should then focus on the most relevant aspects, leaving out details and future steps that do not have to be taken immediately (Voelter et al. 2005). Special attention should also be paid to the therapeutic options the oncologist has to offer; a clear agenda of the next steps and information about the accessibility of medical care at any time will reassure the patient. Asking the patient if there are additional questions and concerns or if she would like to have a significant other to be with her at the next consultation, may close the consultation (Maguire et al. 1996). In other words, information of vulnerable patients should be kept clear and simple and it should be also emphasized that the therapeutic steps are specifically defined and usually well tolerated.

Vulnerable and overwhelmed patients are sometimes confused and ask a lot of questions in an attempt to gain control over the situation; but any additional information, even if it is medically correct and adapted to the questions, may

Table 3 General recommendations for communicating bad news

Provide an adequate setting, which is not disturbed
Be aware of anxiety symptoms, which may hamper communication
Inform about the objectives of the meeting and the time available
Adapt your information to the patient and focus on the essential
Check the patient's understanding and explicitly invite questions
Use also open questions and clarify patient's statements
Avoid early comforting or immediate propositions of "solutions" for psychological distress
Pay attention to non-verbal expressions and other cues from the patient
Communicate your understanding for the patient's experiences and emotions
Allow pauses, name transitions between themes and summarize
Inform about further steps, future meetings and how to be contacted

Table 4 Sources of clinicians' discomfort when breaking bad news

To hurt the patient and being unable to support him
To face painful emotions
To know the fatal outcome and having to withhold this information
To face unrealistic expectations of the patient
To induce high levels of distress or psychiatric disturbances

increase confusion and a feeling of being out of control. When confronted with patients who have a great difficulty to understand the medical condition, oncologists tend to add information which further deteriorates the patient's capacities to regain control. In such situations, a clear leadership by the oncologist is necessary, taking into account the elements listed in Table 2.

Such an approach is more beneficial than persevering in a way that would be adequate for an autonomous patient who is fully able to cope with the situation.

4.2 General Recommendations and Barriers to Adequate Information About a Cancer Diagnosis

For patients who show efficient coping strategies and no signs of important psychological vulnerabilities, communication of a cancer di-

agnosis may be based on recommendations that have been described elsewhere (Maguire 1976; Faulkner and Maguire 1996; Dosanjh et al. 2001; Jenkins and Fallowfield 2002) (see Table 3).

These recommendations are often known but often not followed. Why is it so difficult to break bad news? Disclosure of a cancer diagnosis evokes anxiety in patients, which interferes with their ability to fully understand and follow the explanations. It also evokes anxiety in the oncologist, which interferes with his ability to communicate. Anxiety arises for various reasons. In the following, we will present the main sources of oncologists' discomfort when breaking bad news, and provide some elements which may be of help (Stiefel 2004) (see Table 4).

4.2.1 Fear of Hurting the Patient

One of the main reasons for anxiety when disclosing a cancer diagnosis is the fear to hurt the patient. Since a cancer diagnosis is a major stressor, this fear is justified. The more an oncologist accepts that this news is hurting the patient, the less he has to defend himself and the more authentic he can be. While it is very rare that patients link the bad news to the messenger and hold him responsible, on a less conscious level, the physician–patient relationship is coloured by this fear. To openly address this issue, that "it hurts to hear bad news", is a more adequate way of dealing with the situation than to try to act as if nothing painful happens. An understanding and empathic attitude, legitimating the feelings evoked in the patient, is an effective and sufficient support in such a situation. If the clinician is able to accept that "this is what he can and should do", he might be less haunted by the thought that he is unable to support the patient.

4.2.2 Facing the Patient's Emotions

Another main reason for the oncologist's discomfort when disclosing a cancer diagnosis concerns the patient's emotions. While most of the patients are not yet able to feel or express their emotions at the time of disclosure of a cancer diagnosis, projections of the healthy physician, of what the patient may experience, are frequent. Physicians, like most healthy persons, imagine that the emotional impact of a cancer diagnosis is unbearable; however, experience shows that most cancer patients cope with their situation (Stiefel et al. 2001). Cancer patients may be sad, nervous, irritated, tense or anxious, but these feelings are in the range of normality and are natural steps in the adjustment. As such, they do not have to be treated or alleviated, and the patient does not have such expectations. The only expectations patients may have—and even this is not always the case—is that they wish to express their feelings and that their feelings, even the negative ones, are perceived and acknowledged by the clinicians with empathy. In other words: between imagination and reality, of how an oncologist has to face the patient's emotions, there may be a considerable gap. The ability of clinicians to handle their own painful feelings is closely related to their capacity to contain the patient's feelings; this ability is also coloured by biographical circumstances. Working in oncology entails being able to cope with painful emotions; clinicians who feel that they have difficulties in this area may think of sharing their experiences with peers or attending regular supervisions. It is also the responsibility of senior oncologists to not only transmit technical knowledge, but also to identify young colleagues with difficulties facing emotionally stressful situations and to help them get the help they need.

4.2.3 Patient's Knowledge/ Physician's Knowledge

Another reason for clinicians to feel uncomfortable when disclosing a cancer diagnosis concerns their detailed knowledge about the medical situation, about its unpredictability and sometimes the very bad prognosis. Indeed, it is uncomfortable not to be able to share these thoughts with the patient. Since it is not justified to load the patient with all the possible outcomes, when his energy is needed to fight the cancer, the oncologist has to select information that is most relevant for a given patient at a given moment of the disease. The more the clinician accepts this responsibility, that not all, but only relevant information should be transmitted to the patient, the more he or she will be comfortable with this situation. Of course, whether information is relevant or not, and whether the patient or the clinician is the target of protection, has to be faced with honesty. Not transmitting irrelevant information has to be distinguished from lying, which is consciously withholding relevant information. However, if patients ask specific questions about the disease, they have to be answered correctly, after having clarified why the patient wants to obtain such detailed information and what kind of benefits he expects.

4.2.4 Patient's Expectations

Discomfort and anxiety also arise when facing any unrealistic expectations of the patient. In such situations, it might be difficult to block the patient's "optimism". The statement that there may be limited possibilities may help the oncologist to cope with such a patient, but the pressure may remain at a less conscious level and anxiety may arise, of not being able to fulfil the patient's expectations. When working in oncology, it is often not possible to live up to the expectations of the patients. Almost all patients desire, at least at the time of diagnosis, to be cured. While it is legitimate for a patient to expect to be cured, it does not imply that the progression of the disease is the oncologist's fault. Only very rarely do patients fail to understand that medicine has limits; most of the patients struggle with the fact that they cannot be cured, but are most grateful for their care. Unmet patient expectations are therefore often a problem of the oncologist, especially if they are convinced that the progression of the disease is a personal failure (Stiefel and Guex 1996). Clinicians who consider that cure is a success and palliation a failure are more prone to feel guilty in many situations. A reflection about their own expectations and their professional objectives is therefore necessary to achieve a more mature professional identity.

4.2.5 Other Sources of Discomfort for the Oncology Clinician

Other sources of discomfort concern the fear of inducing a high level of distress and psychiatric disturbances in the patient. This may occur very rarely in vulnerable patients; more often it reflects a projection of the clinician and the wish to "protect" the patient is more related to the clinician's own needs. Unless there are clear indications that a patient is psychologically vulnerable and one has to adapt the information, withholding information is not acceptable. Sometimes patients of a specific cultural background might have different needs with regard to disclosure of diagnosis; in such situations, one has to clarify this issue before proceeding in a standard way. Culturally bound aspects of physician–patient communication are presented in the chapter "Cultural Aspects of Communication in Cancer Care", by A. Surbone, in this volume.

Psychiatric patients are also often a source of distress for oncology clinicians. Generally, there is no need to treat them differently than any other patient, unless there are indications from the patient or from the treating psychiatrist that disclosure has to be adapted. It often happens that information is withheld from psychiatric patients without any reason. Because psychiatric patients, especially those who are subjected to paranoid ideation, are very sensitive and able to catch the essence of a medical situation without explicit communication, they may become tense and mistrusting when they feel that a clinician is withholding information. Discomfort arises in many other situations and is shaped by the bio-

graphical circumstances of the oncology clinician; sometimes, identification with the patient, due to sociodemographic or other variables, hampers adequate communication. Sharing one's own experiences with colleagues, or within a regular supervision, may then be helpful for the clinician and the patient.

4.3 Announcing Relapse

Relapse is associated with deception. What has been hoped and fought for, cure, is no longer possible. Patients might say "But I thought I was cured...", and oncologists might answer, "But I have told you that the chance to be cured was not a hundred percent...". These sentences illustrate the communicational difficulties associated with relapse; possible ways to handle such situations are discussed in the chapter "Key Elements of Communication in Cancer Care", by E. Maex and C. De Valck, in this volume.

4.3.1 Deception, an Inevitable Feeling After Relapse

In the above-mentioned example, both patient and oncologist are right; the patient thought she was cured and the oncologist had told her, at the time of diagnosis, that cure was likely, although not guaranteed. The objective of communicating about relapse is not to know who is right and who is wrong, but to accept how the patient feels, and to acknowledge that the patient's feelings are understandable. Deception does not have to be waved away by providing an optimistic outlook about possible treatments; this would only hamper the clinician's credibility. The patient must first be invited to express this deception, and he has the right to hear that his feelings are understandable. It is also important to understand that patients' statements such as "I've had enough, I'm not interested in further treatment" have to be perceived less as an information and more as an expression of an emotional state. Such statements do not need to be immediately contradicted by scientifico-medical arguments, nor do they have to be negotiated. Allowing a moment of decep-

Table 5 Key elements of communication when facing relapse

Acknowledge the deception associated with relapse and allow time to accept the bad news
Do not deny patient's current experience, try to understand what he/she goes through
Avoid premature comforting or an immediate focus on further therapeutic strategies
Understand pessimistic patients' statements as transient expressions of discouragement
Introduce nuances in extreme point of views ("all or nothing" statements)
Explicitly inform that there is choice and that refusal of further treatment is an option
Welcome ambivalence about future treatments as an adequate reaction after relapse
Inform that new treatments can be questioned later at any time
Support also patients who make—from a medical point of view—an unreasonable choice

tion or irritation, before addressing the possible benefits of further treatments, is therefore a more appropriate way of facing relapse with a patient (see Table 5).

4.3.2 Introducing Nuances in a Traumatising Situation

After deception has been expressed and acknowledged by the clinician in an empathic way, the next step is to communicate that such situations are often perceived as traumatising and that nuances may, for a moment, be lost. The law of "all or nothing" may dominate and thoughts such as "Let's give it up", "I will not go through other treatments again" or "This is all hopeless and senseless" may occur. It might take some time, and the clinician is well advised to provide the necessary time, until the patient is able again to integrate the new situation, before being ready to continue treatment.

4.3.3 Overcoming Feelings of Impotence/ The Competent Patient

The decision to initiate new treatments after relapse has to be taken by the patient. In order to face a new series of treatments, it is necessary that the patient expresses his or her readiness to enter a new treatment phase. An important element in overcoming the first feelings of impotence after relapse is to perceive that there is a choice. Indeed, a patient may or may not accept a new treatment line. Choice is a powerful tool to overcome feelings of impotence; this is one of the reasons why this choice has to be left to the patient and why clinicians should not present the situation as if there is only one option. Not only from a psychological point of view, but also from a legal and ethical point of view, the patient has the right to refuse further treatments. In order to present this choice to the patient in an adequate way, the clinician first has to accept that there is such a choice and that there are patients who may refuse a treatment, even if this seems, from a medical point of view, to be the wrong decision. As long as patients are competent, they have the right to choose. Unfortunately, there is still confusion about competency of the patient and there are still clinicians who believe that a patient is incompetent if he or she makes decisions which are unreasonable from a medical point of view, or if he or she suffers from psychiatric disturbances; both situations are not a proof of incompetence (Markson et al.1994). Clinicians who ignore these facts and who are ambivalent about patients refusing treatment are at risk of breaking the laws when putting pressure on patients to continue treatments. They are also counterproductive from a psychological point of view, since they deny the choice of the patient and enhance feelings of "being treped" and feelings of impotence.

4.3.4 Building a Therapeutic Alliance

Once the patient is able to decide about further treatments, their benefits and possible risks should be discussed and the patient should be informed that he has the right change his mind, when he considers the benefits do not outweigh the side effects. Too often a new treatment line is introduced and there is no discussion about how the patient feels about it. Bitterness of having paid a too heavy price might then occur if the treatment fails to respond to the expectations. Because of fear that the patient refuses a medically reasonable treatment, clinicians often encourage the patient by minimizing its side effects. Such an attitude evokes in the patients a feeling of isolation and hampers the therapeutic alliance, which is most important during the progression of disease. On the contrary, if the clinician is sensitive to the patient's ambivalence, which is an adequate feeling towards the introduction of further treatments after relapse, he is perceived as a careful and competent professional and as a trustful partner. If a patient refuses further treatments, guilt about this decision (for example towards significant others) should not be increased by making the patient feel that he has made an unreasonable choice.

Oncology clinicians also have to accept a patient who is not complying with medical propositions. Such propositions may be reasonable from a medical point of view, but unacceptable for the patient from a psychological point of view. There is no hierarchy between body and mind, and no hierarchy between physician and patient when it comes to making decisions about further treatments. A clinical vignette can illustrate this point.

A 38-year-old patient suffering from chronic paranoid schizophrenia was referred to consultation liaison psychiatry after his refusal to continue palliative treatment of a testicular cancer, known to respond to chemotherapy. Upon evaluation, the patient appeared competent with regard to medical treatment decisions; he understood the situation, knew the treatment options and their outcomes and explained his refusal to continue treatment by the fact that each treatment and contact with the medical staff was associated with unbearable anxiety, despite an adequate psychopharmacological treatment. He had informed his son, a teenager, that he would not accept any further treatment, that he knew that he would die of the disease in the near future and told him how much he loved him and how sad he was of not having been able to share these feelings with him because of his mental illness. In conclusion, he told the psychiatrist, "You know doctor, I prefer to die physically than go through hell mentally again ...".

While other patients may be ready to pay a heavy physical and psychological price to prolong their lives, this patient clearly indicated that for him psychological suffering has reached its limits. After an in-depth discussion, his wish was respected and he was comforted in his decision.

4.4 Informing About Progression and Prognosis of Disease

Progression of disease is another crucial moment in the physician–patient communication. When progression occurs, patients—sometimes for the first time—are preoccupied with the outcome of their disease. This preoccupation may be explicitly expressed or communicated in an indirect way by means of projects or questions which concern the near future. However, for other patients, progression of disease does not seem to be preoccupying at all. The two scenarios will be discussed in the section that follows.

4.4.1 Denial and Progression of Disease

Sometimes a patient appears more optimistic or indifferent when progression of disease occurs. This is most often due to denial. In such a situation, it might be wise to wait for cues from the patient, which provide an occasion to inform him about medical facts. Therefore, the clinician should underline from time to time that the medical situation is serious and—if the patient then wants to know more—initiate a careful discussion. This recommendation is based on the rule that a patient copes if she can, denies if she must and becomes psychotic if she is forced to (Weisman 1979). A clinical vignette illustrates this point.

A 40-year-old woman with small children who suffered from advanced breast cancer showed an important degree of anxiety as soon as her medical diagnosis was discussed; in such moments, she tried to change the topic, indicating that she knew enough about her disease and that she did not wish to obtain additional information. Despite her indications that she was unwilling or unable to hear more about the disease, the treating physician insisted on repeatedly explaining to her in detail the state of her condition. As he stated, this was in his opinion the only way that the woman could start a mourning process, which would finally lead her to accept the disease and the fatal outcome. After first trying to avoid these confrontations, the patient then responded that she didn't know what the physician was talking about and that she was feeling quite well. A day later, she told the medical staff that someone died during the night in the hospital room; this was not the case. Only half an hour later, she pulled out her intravenous lines, rushed to the floor and cried "They kill people in this hospital, they want to intoxicate me ... ". The patient was physically contained, and a neuroleptic was injected; within seconds and before the medication could have an effect, she calmed down and stated: "I know that you don't want to hurt me, I am just terribly anxious about my disease".

This example illustrates that a brief psychotic episode was induced by not respecting this patient's inability to accept the unbearable thought of having to die and to leave her small children alone. Her paranoid imagination of intoxication may be understood as the psychologically intoxicating "information practice" of the treating physician.

4.4.2 Discussing Progression and Prognosis

Most patients, at one moment or another, would like to know their condition when progression occurs. Questions about prognosis of disease can be answered in different ways—one way is to avoid the question by stating that predicting outcome is very difficult in oncology, and another is to provide statistical information, which indicates a medium survival time in months. This later attitude often does not meet the needs of the patient but the needs of the physician so as to get rid of the problem. A patient-centred way to answer such questions is to try to understand the preoccupations of the patients and what they

Table 6 Informing about progression and prognosis of disease

Try to pick up patients' cues concerning preoccupations about the future
Ask the patient about the aspects and degree of details he/she wishes to know
Avoid contradictory information, assure interdisciplinary agreement
Maintain hope without denying the seriousness of the medical situation
Respect denial and inform significant others about its protecting function
Schedule regular follow-up visits and invite the patient to maintain contact

think about the current condition, before exploring what kind of information they would like to receive. While there are patients who feel more in control by obtaining detailed medical information, others like to know if cure or delaying the progression is still possible, without asking questions about what will happen later.

Discussing progression of disease also includes information about the future (see Table 6).

In this phase of the illness it is especially important that the patient receives the same message from all staff members in order to enhance a feeling of coherence and to prevent confusion. This topic is presented in the chapter "Interdisciplinary Communication", by F. Porchet, in this volume. Since progression of disease represents a considerable psychological distress, measures that counteract patient feelings of abandonment are necessary. Beside the trusting relationship a clinician has established with the patient, regular follow-up visits and an invitation to call if there are concerns are beneficial.

4.5 Communication with the Terminal Cancer Patient

Since communication with the terminally ill is covered in the chapter "Maintaining Hope: Communication in Palliative Care" (by V. Kennedy and M. Lloyd-Williams), this section will be restricted to a few thoughts on the situation of the dying patient (Guex et al. 2000).

Due to exhaustion and a certain withdrawal of patients when facing the end of their life, communication with the treating physician is often limited to short conversations. Communication is less dominated by the transmission of specific medical information. More often, non-verbal communication and therefore the attitude of the clinician becomes crucial. He has to contain the patient's suffering: communication should then not be restricted to medical facts, and trying to cover up the unpleasant aspects of the situation is inadequate. If a physician wants to be open to understand "where a patient is at a given moment", he has to free himself from prejudices of how someone has to face death. While in prior stages of the disease, the clinician often plays an active role, in the terminal phase, he is invited to listen and to try to understand the patient; he is in a more "receptive" position.

A 28-year-old man of Italian origin, suffering from a very advanced lymphoma, used to ask the treating physician every morning during rounds, "Is there a possibility to operate?" and would then change the topic and inform the physician about the latest news from the Italian football league. The physician always respectfully denied a surgical option for that moment and then stayed a while to listen to the football news.

Being with the patient "where he is at this moment in time" implied that the daily question of this patient was respectfully answered without irritation, and understood in the context of the patient's denial. This question, which had become a ritual, was this patient's way to express that he knew he is ill, but that he had not given up hope; the football news can be interpreted as the patient expressing that he is not only ill, but that healthy parts still exist and that he continues to be interested in his lifelong hobby, which he shared with the physician.

Being close to the patient also means including the family; very often clinicians can enhance the understanding of significant others, that each patient has the right to die his own death and that the most important and active task family members have is to be close to the patient and respect his way of coping with the situation. The key elements of communicating with the family are discussed in the chapter "The Patient and His Family", by P. Firth.

4.6 Conclusions

We have tried to discuss the key elements of communication in crucial moments over the course of disease. Each of these moments requires a careful attention to the specific challenges they represent for the cancer patient and the treating physician. Some communication skills that clinicians acquire during their professional life are due to their increased experiences, feeling more secure and less anxious over time; other skills are based on theoretical knowledge of the patient–physician communication and on a reflection on their own expectations, fears and attitudes, regarding their roles as health care professionals. But certainly one of the most beneficial ways to improve communication is to participate in the emerging communication skills training, which is based on interactivity, role plays and video- or audio-analyses of interviews with simulated patients. This communication skills training is described in the chapters "Current Concepts of Communication Skills Training in Oncology" and "Communication Skills Training in Oncology: It Works!".

References

1. Berney A, Stiefel F (2004) Psychiatric symptoms. In: Voltz R, Bernat JL, Borasio GD, Maddocks I, Oliver D, Portenoy RK (eds) Palliative care in neurology. Oxford University Press, New York, pp 272–279
2. Bragard I, Razavi D, Marchal S et al. (2006) Teaching communication and stress management skills. Support Care Cancer (2006) 14:454–461
3. Delvaux N, Merckaert I, Marchal S et al. (2005) Physicians' communication with a cancer patient and a relative: a randomized study assessing the efficacy of consolidation workshops. Cancer 103:2397–2411
4. Dosanjh S, Barnes J, Bhandari M (2001) Barriers to breaking bad news among medical and surgical residents [see comment]. Medical Education 35:197–205

5. Faulkner A, Maguire P (1996) Talking to cancer patients and their relatives. Oxford University Press, New York

6. Guex P, Stiefel F, Rousselle I (2000) Psychotherapy with Patients with Cancer 230. Psychother Rev 2:269–273

7. Jenkins V, Fallowfield L (2002) Can communication skills training alter physicians' beliefs and behavior in clinics? J Clin Oncol 20:765–769

8. Maguire P, Faulkner A, Booth K, Elliott C, Hillier V (1996) Helping cancer patients disclose their concerns. Eur J Cancer 32A:78–81

9. Markson LJ, et al. (1994) Physician assessment of patient competence. J Am Geriatr Soc 42:1074–1080

10. Razavi D, Stiefel F (1994) Common psychiatric disorders in cancer patients. I. Adjustment disorders and depressive disorders. Support Care Cancer 2:223–232

11. Razavi D, Merckaert I, Marchal S et al. (2003) How to optimize physicians' communication skills in cancer care: results of a randomized study assessing the usefulness of posttraining consolidation workshops. J Clin Oncol 21:3141–3149

12. Stiefel F, Razavi D (1994) Common psychiatric disorders in cancer patients. II. Anxiety and acute confusional states. Support Care Cancer 2:233–237

13. Stiefel F, Guex P (1996) Palliative and supportive care: At the frontier of medical omnipotence. Ann Oncol 7:135–138

14. Stiefel F, Die Trill M, Berney A, Olarte J, Razavi D (2001) Depression in palliative care: a pragmatic report from the Expert Working Group of the European Association for Palliative Care. Support Care Cancer 9:477–788

15. Stiefel F (2004) La communication médecin-malade : éléments clés. Médecine & Hygiène 62:57

16. Voelter V, Mirimanoff RO, Stiefel F, Rousselle I, Leyvraz S (2005) L'annonce d'une mauvaise nouvelle en oncologie. Revue Médicale Suisse 20:1350–1353

17. Weisman A (1979) Coping with cancer. McGraw-Hill, Book Company ed. New York

5 Maintaining Hope: Communication in Palliative Care

V. Kennedy, M. Lloyd-Williams

Recent Results in Cancer Research, Vol. 168
© Springer-Verlag Berlin Heidelberg 2006

5.1 Introduction

From "What's Left", by Kerry Hardie'

I know more or less
How to live my life now.
But I want to know how to live what's left
With my eyes open and my hands open;
I want to stand at the door in the rain
Listening, sniffing, gaping.
Fearful and joyous,
Like an idiot before God.

Good communication between healthcare professionals is crucial within palliative care. Many have found that good communication can lead to a greater sense of well-being, decreasing feelings of distress commonly experienced by those diagnosed with a terminal illness and their families.

Much of the literature related to communication often is related to "information" and about "telling the truth". It is important to note, however, that communicating this type of information and/or news alone may not result in effective communication. How and when this information/discussion is offered is an important factor in how a patient may respond to it.

5.2 The Importance of Communication in Palliative Care

Psychological and psychiatric morbidity is a common problem for cancer patients as well as their carers, relatives and friends, and depression has been found to be especially common for those people with advanced cancer. It has been suggested that 25%–50% of patients suffer from psychological distress (Fallowfield et al. 2001) and it has been further found that the risk of experiencing depression is increased when the disease is advanced (Breitbart 1995; Fallowfield et al. 2001), or when functional impairment or symptoms are greater (Hopwood and Stephens 2000). A systematic review by Hotopf et al. (2002) found that depression is a very common problem in palliative care patients, but that many of the studies in this area were lacking, and "based on small samples of patients with very high non-participation rates". Diagnosis and treatment of psychological distress and disturbance, however, is based on communication.

Indeed, one aspect thought to help patient and family distress includes effective and open communication with health professionals. Communication has been said to be important for patient understanding of their disease, outcomes, patient behaviour, ability to cope, both physical and psychological health, as well as patient satisfaction with care, and compliance with treatment.

Research have found that many patients want as much detailed information as possible about their illness and treatment, and want to be part of the decision-making process (Kirk et al. 2004). In a study by Sapir et al. (2000) of 103 cancer patients, they found that 92% would want to know all the information. They also found that the oncologist was the staff member most often sought out for both information and support. Furthermore, Kirk et al. (2004) in 72 participants registered with palliative care in Canada and Australia found that all patients wanted information about their illness, and wanted it fully shared with relatives. Moody (2003) also describes the great need of cancer patients for information, and for the appropriate information at the appropriate time. The literature demonstrates that good information can help patients in decision-making, and with psychological and physical well-being (Greenwood 2002).

Although many have reported the importance of communication, the literature has also shown that patients do not receive the appropriate information (Kutner et al. 1999; Ong et al. 1995) and/or that the information given is poor (Lo and Snyder 1999). However, a study by Sapir et al. (2000) found that 85% of their participants were satisfied with the clarity of the information they received and 90% thought it was given to them sensitively. Aspects of social desirability which may influence these results, have to be taken into account for interpretation of such studies. Although patients may be well informed about diagnosis, treatment, and prognosis, there is less coverage of psychological and well-being issues with the patient (Ford et al. 1996).

It has been said that the withholding of information from patients regarding their illness and treatment is mostly due to doctor "intuition", which has also been said to be incorrect in most cases (Fallowfield 1997; Husebo 1998). Whereas in previous years withholding information to protect patients, and not to diminish hope, was common practice, more recently truth telling has become the more common practice (Nekolaichuk and Bruera 1998). Although a move to a more open awareness from a more closed awareness has been identified over the years, Field and Copp (1999) additionally describe a further move in the 1990s to a more "conditional awareness", particularly in palliative care where they say health professionals are more likely to give "graduated dosages of truth" (Field and Copp 1999).

It is believed that many physicians/healthcare professionals limit the information they give to their patients and family in order to try and spare them what might be bad news; however,

research has demonstrated that this can actually cause greater difficulties for individuals by not allowing them to plan for the future (Fallowfield et al. 2002).

Further suggestions as to why communication between doctor and patient (health professionals and patients) is less than optimal include lack of time and differences between knowledge, values, expectations, and goals (Cantwell and Ramirez 1997; Friedrichsen et al. 2000). In most of Northern Europe and North America patients are now regularly informed about their cancer diagnosis and prognosis (to the best of the physician's capability), but in countries such as Eastern Europe, Spain, and South America such issues are rarely discussed with patients and their families, demonstrating possible cultural differences between communication needs and/or attitudes (Bruera et al. 2000). Bruera and co-workers (2000) did find a significant regional difference in patterns of practice regarding communication at the end of life, emphasising again the need for individualised communication strategies.

Communication is said to be even more difficult and more important for those with a terminal illness or when care changes from curative to palliative (Friedrichsen et al. 2000; Kutner et al. 1999). Open communication is an important aspect of death and dying and of a "good death", and it is thought to contribute to effective symptom control and end of life planning (Edmonds and Rogers 2003; Field and Copp 1999).

However, research suggests that these needs are not being met, and that many physicians and nurses do not discuss care with patients at the end of life, and even when they do they may not talk about such issues as concerns or fears (Addington-Hall et al. 1995; Edmonds and Rogers 2003; Lo and Snyder 1999). Cantwell and Ramirez (1997) found that only 21% of their participants (junior house officers) asked dying patients about any emotional concerns. Nurses also focus on physical care, avoiding open communication about prognosis and other psychological and spiritual issues (Edmonds and Rogers 2003; Rogers et al. 2000).

5.3 Role of Health Professionals: What Can Professionals Do?

Conversations about end of life with patients and families are never easy; however, physicians need to have such discussions in order to benefit the patient (Lo and Snyder 1999). The importance of providing honest information has been described in the previous section, outlining the importance of telling the "truth" to patients about their illness, treatment, as well as prognosis.

In addition to telling the truth, using appropriate language is also fundamental in communicating with patients and their family (Fallowfield et al. 2002). It is important to use unambiguous language and to make sure that the patient understands what has been said. It is not uncommon for patients to leave the consultation without having fully understood what has been said (Fallowfield et al. 2002; Quirt et al. 1997).

Ong et al. (1995) describe two types of physician behaviour whilst communicating with patients: instrumental and affective. Instrumental behaviour describes "cure-oriented" behaviour that is "task oriented", and affective behaviour describes "care-oriented" behaviour that is "socio-emotional". Friedrichsen et al. (2000) found that there were many different types of physicians, for example (1) the inexperienced messenger, (2) the emotionally burdened, (3) the rough and ready expert, (4) the benevolent but tactless expert, (5) the distanced doctor and (6) the empathic professional. They found that the character of the physicians and their ability to create personal relationships also influence the patients' ability to cope with the situation and with the information given to them.

There is no consensus on what may be considered to be the best form of communicating (Friedrichsen et al. 2000). Physicians who are able to empathise and care—as well as provide hope, trust, interest and commitment—are important to patients, as is allowing the patient and family the opportunity to ask questions (Friedrichsen et al 2000). In addition, using non-verbal as well as verbal communication has been considered important, particularly in re-enforcing messages (Fallowfield et al. 2002).

Some have suggested methods that may help in communication with dying patients particularly with regards to breaking bad news, including Fallowfield (1993), Faulkner and colleagues (1995), Morton (1996), and Girgis (1998), for example.

Maintaining open communication between health professionals and patient may, however, not be as easy in practice as it may appear on paper (Field and Copp 1999). Bolmsjo and Hermenen (1998) describe a situation where a person's response to health professionals can change from time to time, making it less clear what form of communication may be most appropriate at each stage.

Although much of what has been described so far relates to doctor–patient communication, nurse–patient communication is also very important to consider, although it has received much less attention in the literature to date. Kruijver et al. (2000) highlight effective communication behaviours by nurses in cancer care. Behaviours thought to be facilitating effective communication by nurses included empathy, touch, comforting and supportive care behaviours. They confirm Raudonis's, (1993) finding that "empathic relationships between nurses and hospice patients had a positive impact on patients' physical and emotional well-being" (Kruijver et al. 2000). Morales (1994) found that touch is important in transmitting confidence and in enhancing the patient's ability to cope and feel accepted as a person (Kruijver et al. 2000; Morales 1994). Bottorff et al. (1995) reported that comfort involves more than pain relief but that it also includes "humour, physical comfort, emotionally supportive statements, and comforting and connecting touch" (Kruijver et al. 2000). Kruijver and co-workers (2000) believe that the types of behaviours described above can contribute to helping or hindering patients in expressing their informational needs or concerns, as well as affecting their satisfaction with care.

In their study of 103 cancer patients, Sapir et al. (2000) found that 87% felt that eye contact was important, 53% were strongly in favour of having the doctor sitting across the desk, while 38% felt strongly in favour of having the doctor sitting next to them. Supportive touch had as many in favour as it had against, with 15% having a strong disapproval to this.

Communicating news, particularly regarding transferring from curative to palliative care, is very stressful for physicians and health professionals, and many are often left unsatisfied with their consultation (Fallowfield et al. 2002). For this reason it is also important to consider the needs not only of the patient and their family who are receiving the information, but also of those individuals who are providing the information. Fallowfield et al. (2002), for example, express a need for adequate support for health professionals working in this area to help deal with such stressful situations.

Since communication has been identified as an important aspect of palliative care, and since it has been found that health professionals, e.g. physicians and/or nurses, have been less than optimal (Kruijver et al. 2000; Lo and Snyder 1999), education in this area has increased in the last decade. The effectiveness of such communication skills programmes has been supported by some authors (Wilkinson et al. 1998).

Although honest communication and information is wanted by both patients and their family and friends, it is also important to consider that their needs may differ in nature to some degree. Field and Copp (1999) suggest that patients and relatives face different threats, "relatives have to cope with bereavement, whereas the dying patient has to face the end of their existence, and for them there may be the need to escape into the comfort of mental avoidance and/or denial of the outcome".

In terms of the content of communication, two important areas described by Kirk et al. (2004) were those of prognosis and of hope. The participants in this study described a great need for hope and to be given "hopeful messages at all stages". The authors go on to describe two dimensions of hope that are relevant. The first, "patient/family orientations to hope", involves needing to believe in a miracle and living parallel realities—that is, hoping for a cure or remission whilst at the same time realising the terminal nature of the illness. The second dimension of hope described involved "messages from the healthcare providers supporting hope" including using words and approaches that left the door open,

retained professional honesty, pacing the move towards palliative care, and respecting alternative paths (Kirk et al. 2004).

The importance of hope as part of effective communication is described clearly in this study; however, the importance of hope is not by far limited to this one study. Many have described hope as a crucial aspect of communication within palliative care patients and their families. The following section will explore the role and importance of hope as a major aspect of communication in palliative care.

5.4   Hope

Some might think that the last place to expect to find "hope" would be in those with a terminal illness. Many of those working within palliative care, however, will be aware of the importance of hope to those who are facing an uncertain future. Research (Herth and Cutcliffe 2002; Penson 2000) concludes that hope is an important aspect of palliative care, and therefore of communication within palliative care. The importance of maintaining hope within palliative care may be essential to the well-being of the patient an/or family; however, being able to provide hope may be a challenging task for health professionals concerned.

The following section aims to give a brief account of what hope may encompass for individuals, specifically for those receiving palliative care. We will then consider the literature with regards to the benefits for patients in maintaining hope at the later stages of life, and finally we will discuss the role of the health professional in maintaining hope and the ways in which this can be done in communication.

5.5   What Is Hope?

The aim of this section is not to provide a comprehensive review of the philosophical history of "hope", but to consider hope in the context of palliative care, and what it means to those individuals with a terminal illness.

In the literature hope has often been related to the spiritual and physical being, as well as to coping with difficult situations (Chaplin and Mc-Intyre 2001; Herth and Cutcliffe 2002). And although there may be many perspectives on hope, Chaplin and McIntyre (2001) state that there is a:

"General acceptance that hope is multidimensional in character and dynamic in nature and that it provides an energising force which allows individuals to cope with their current life situation and also provides the opportunity for personal growth" (p. 119).

Hope has been described as something that allows people to think about death and life after death without "entering into utter despair" (Cutcliffe and Herth 2002), and as something "to be present in all stages of life, including dying" (Cutcliffe 1995). It appears therefore that hope may be something of great relevance to those who are terminally ill.

With respect to palliative care in particular, hope has become an increasingly important aspect of care and research (Herth and Cutcliffe 2002). Although much of research available for palliative care is with respect to cancer patients (Chaplin and McIntyre 2001), some authors have studied hope in relation to other illnesses such as HIV or motor neuron disease (Hall 1990; Rabkin et al. 1990; Silani and Borasio 1999). Hall (1990) stated that "it is just as important to have hope in the hour before one's death as it is to have hope in other stages of one's life".

As for what hope means for those within palliative care, there have been some attempts in the literature at definitions. Dufault and Martoocchio (1985) studied hope in patients with cancer, and in doing so identified two types of hope: particularised and generalised hope. They described particularised hope as being linked with a specific goal, such as improvement in health, while generalised hope was not linked to a particular object (Dufault and Martoocchio 1985; Nekolaichuk and Bruera 1998). And for cancer patients specifically, Dufault and Martoocchio (1985) defined hope as:

"A multidimensional dynamic life force characterised by a confident yet uncertain expectation of achieving a future good which, to the hoping per-

son, is realistically possible and personally significant" (Dufault and Martocchio 1985).

In 1989, Owen studied nurses perspectives on the meaning of hope in cancer patients. Based on her study she developed a model that has six dimensions which included (1) goal setting, (2) positive personal attributes, (3) future redefinition, (4) meaning in life, (5) peace and (6) energy. From this she defined hope as "a dynamic process in which patients respond to changing life events" (Owen 1989).

Herth in 1990 studied hope more specifically in the terminally ill and found that for this group hope was described as:

"An inner power directed toward a new awareness and enrichment of 'being' rather than 'rational expectations'" (Herth 1990; p. 1257).

More recently, Flemming (1997), in a phenomenological study of four participants, explained the meaning of hope to palliative care cancer patients. He found that areas influential in maintaining hope included (a) control of disease progression underpinned by a hope for cure; (b) positive interest in the individual by doctors and nurses by "being there"; and (c) third and most important was the presence of family members, and the anticipated future with them. Loosing control over any of the above factors was further identified as a cause for loss of hope.

For patients within palliative care it has also been said that hope is associated with more than just hope for cure, and that patients develop different "goal-directed hopes" such as "hope for cure, hope for relief from pain, hope to accomplish a specific task before dying, hope for a peaceful death" (Nekolaichuk and Bruera 1998).

Benzein and Saveman (1998) studied nurses' perspectives of hope in patients with cancer, and found that nurses had problems defining hope in a simple way, but expressed it as a "realistic and future-oriented phenomenon". Hope was found to be related to inner strength and energy, significant events, support from relatives and staff, and/or familiar environment, confidence in medical treatment, and nursing actions and treatments. Their results highlighted the importance of a good relationship with staff.

5.5.1 "Benefits" of Hope

Hope has been said to be associated with a good sense of well-being and psychological state, decreasing distress and stress, as well as increasing coping ability, and having a positive effect on physical health. Stephenson (1991), for example, describes how hope in healthcare has been described as a factor in maintaining and regaining health, as well as in helping a person to accept limitations and death.

Benzein and Saveman (1998) in their paper refer to studies that have shown that when a person looses hope, negative results can emerge such as apathy, inactivity, meaninglessness, and hopelessness. Lack of hope or "hopelessness", on the other hand, has been associated with negative effects on physical health, depression, and suicidal ideation (Breitbart et al. 2000). In fact, Chaplin and McIntyre (2001) state that "there is evidence to suggest that the total absence of hope within an individual can produce a state of despair that can lead to inevitable death".

For those with a terminal illness, however, maintaining hope in the face of physical, social, psychological and/or spiritual challenges can be very difficult (Chaplin and McIntyre 2001). And in light of what have been found to be significant benefits of hope to a dying individual, it is the duty of those health professionals concerned to do what they can to help maintain hope, to promote holistic care, and to maximise physical, social, psychological, and spiritual health, in the true nature of palliative care.

Cutcliffe (1995) refers to Lynch (1965), who suggested that "hope cannot sustain the individual indefinitely"; hope needs nurturing and feeding by "help" from outside agencies and they both emphasise that due to this hope is a crucial part of nursing.

5.5.2 How Can Health Professionals Help?

A study of 248 cancer patients by Moadel et al. (1999) found that 41% of their participants expressed a need for help in finding hope. Professionals can help maintain hope in various ways which are all ultimately related to communication.

Fanslow (1981) described four phases to help maintain hope in a dying individual, which included cure, treatment, prolongation of life, and peaceful death. She believes that a dying person's hope will evolve through each phase, and she states that "anyone can live with the fact that he has an incurable disease, but no one can live with the thought that he, as a person, is hopeless". These four phases of hope have implications for care, for example, by using appropriate and nonthreatening terminology in the "cure" phase, or by providing spiritual care or company for those in the "peaceful death" phase.

Cutcliffe (1995), by interviewing nurses, examined how they inspire and instil hope in terminally ill HIV patients. They found that staff may do this by "means of an integrated theoretical framework of four key elements or core variables. This is achieved by nursing the person in totality within the context of a formed partnership, underpinned by the affirmation of the individual's worth, which is assured by the nurse entering into the process of reflection in action".

Herth (1990) found in a study of 30 terminally ill adults that nurses can foster hope by supporting/providing interpersonal connectedness (such as being present), attainable aims (by providing guidance in refocusing aims, for example), spiritual comfort (such as praying and receiving visits from members of faith community); lightheartedness, recalling of uplifting memories, and affirmation of worth. Hope-hindering factors included isolation and abandonment, uncontrollable pain and discomfort, and devaluation of personhood.

Koopmeiners et al. (1997) found in their study of 32 people receiving active or supportive treatment or palliative care for cancer that health professionals can influence hope both positively and negatively. The patients in their study identified healthcare professionals who contributed to their hope, in order, as doctors, nurses, chaplains, social workers, other staff, dietician, volunteers, housekeeper, and receptionist. They also found that hope was facilitated by being present and taking time to talk, giving information in a sensitive, compassionate manner and answering questions, and when health professionals demonstrated caring behaviours such as being friendly, nice, or polite. They found negative influences on hope to mainly include ways of how information was given. Poor communication such as being cold, mean, candid, or disrespectful had a negative impact on hope, as did conflicting information between healthcare professionals. Their findings again have direct implications for practice.

Benzein and Saveman (1998) found that if patients encountered a positive attitude from the staff, it would support their hope, whilst absence of nursing presence could contribute to diminishing hope. They believe that nurses can, via their actions and treatment, foster patients' inner strength and energy by using "hope-inspiring" factors such as achieving significant goals and being present on the ward, giving support.

Back et al. (2003) state that by focusing on hope, preparation for the worst may have its downfall, and they suggest that adopting a more "hope for the best, and prepare for the worst" attitude may be most appropriate. They believe that focusing solely on hope (for a cure) may leave the patient "unaware of their limited life expectancy", and may possibly result in missed opportunities to put affairs in order (considered as an important aspect of a good death), and to improve symptom and pain management, as well as to discuss underlying issues such as psychological and/or spiritual issues, for example. Back and colleagues (2003), however, refer to hope mainly in the context of "hoping for a cure", while we have found that hope means more than this for those with a terminal illness, and that in contrast to Back et al., maintaining hope is connected to positive impacts on those psychological, spiritual and existential issues mentioned above.

Penson (2000) says that " acknowledging that hope is not a promise means we have nothing to fear in encouraging it", and suggests that by offering appropriate climate, comfort, communication, and attitude to change for patients can help in fostering hope. She suggests that a hopeful climate can be achieved by recognising the patient's "intrinsic worth", and that comfort can be provided by touch and by securing optimal physical care. Communication is seen as important, being open to listen and to ask questions is crucial in

maintaining hope, and Penson suggests information should be given in a way that is "not unduly negative or falsely reassuring", supporting Back's "hope for the best, and prepare for the worst". This is believed to allow patients to put their affairs in order without feeling as if they are "giving up", lifting a weight and allowing them to enjoy the time that is left. According to Penson, communicating about change is also important in maintaining hope, so that a person can "shift from dying from a terminal illness to living with a life-threatening illness" (Wilkinson 1996).

McIntyre and Chaplin (2001) suggest a conceptual model of hope that can be applied to practice, which incorporates three key themes that are comfort, worth, and attachment. They use this model to demonstrate hope-sustaining and hope-diminishing aspects that may be influenced by health professionals. For comfort, they have identified physical ease as hope sustaining, and physical discomfort as hope diminishing; for attachment, caring relationships have been described as hope sustaining, and abandonment and isolation as hope diminishing; for worth, feeling valued has been thought as hope sustaining, and feeling devalued as hope diminishing. Whilst emphasising the interconnectedness of the model and its themes, they believe this model can be applied to practice, and they provide some hope-sustaining interventions in palliative care based on its principles. See Table 1 for these interventions.

Patients and families have expressed a need for information and truth telling, and as a result telling the truth as opposed to withholding information is currently the most common form of practice, particularly in Western Europe and North America. However, it is crucial to consider how information is given, and it is thought important that it is given with an additional consideration for hope, since it has been suggested that how information is shared can affect a person's experience of hope (Nekolaichik and Bruera 1998), and that breaking bad news by providing "truth without any hope", or "hope without any truth" may be as destructive as each other (Nekolaichuk and Bruera 1998). With respect to telling the truth, Nekolaichik and Bruera (1998) therefore recognise the need to balance truth telling

Table 1 Hope-nurturing interventions in palliative care (from McIntyre and Chaplin 2001)

Theme	Interventions	Rationale
Comfort Aim: to promote physical ease	Comprehensively assess/regularly re-assess pain and other symptoms and implement appropriate interventions promptly Explore psychosocial impact of pain and other symptoms Provide high-quality care to promote comfort (personal and environmental)	To prevent/effectively manage physical and psychosocial distress
Attachment Aim: to promote caring relationships	"Be there" for patient and family when support is needed especially when redefining goals and expectations Provide a friendly, caring environment which recognises the patient's individuality and needs Use humour and discussion of "normal" topics when appropriate Promote communication and privacy between patients and loved ones to facilitate expressions of caring Show concern and caring for the family's needs	Demonstrate caring, confirm value and promote some sense of normality. Facilitate supportive relationships
Worth Aim: to confirm the patient's value to self and others	Explore patient's previous experiences and perceptions of illness Enhance independence utilising appropriate personnel, aids and resources Explore wishes for future e.g. desired place of death and promote decision making Facilitate life review—share personal and family memories Sensitively explore spiritual/religious beliefs and provide support as appropriate	Affirm worth by respecting individuality, promoting autonomy, and respecting beliefs

and hope, as opposed to placing a primary emphasis on truth telling alone. Penson (2000) says that near the end of life, hope needs to be based "not on false promises but on the belief rewarding times can still be had".

Maintaining hope in palliative care patients, however, is not a one-off event; it is a process stretching the length of the individual's remaining life. The ongoing nature of maintaining hope in palliative care patients has been identified by research that describes how hope changes and fluctuates over time within palliative care (Chaplin and McIntyre 2001; Cutcliffe 1995; Flemming 1997; Herth 1993; Hockley 1993). This changing nature of hope reflects the changing nature of the illness, and therefore a demand for an ongoing process of maintaining hope through communication.

It is also important to recognise that is not only the illness and the communication with health professionals that can influence an individual's sense of hope. People and environments surrounding individuals have also been seen to influence levels of hope (Chaplin and McIntyre 2001). This means that such factors will also need to be taken into account when considering the well-being and sense of hope of palliative care patients.

5.5.3 Hope for the Family and Significant Others

Within palliative care, hope should also be considered for those who are close to the patients either personally or professionally. Caring for someone close can be very stressful and has been associated with causing psychological and social distress in carers, and therefore with caregiver burden (Kissane et al. 1997; Pitceathly and Maguire 2003; Siegel et al. 1991).

In terms of psychological effects on the carer,

Pitceathly and Maguire (2003) found, in their review of the psychological impacts of cancer on patients' partners and other key relatives, that most people can cope with the role of caregiver, but that there are an important few that become highly distressed or develop an affective disorder. Farran et al. (1991) suggested that hope was one of the important factors in supporting the ability of carers to cope with the care-giving role under difficult circumstances.

The importance of hope to families and caregivers alike has been supported in other research (Herth 1993; Hickey 1990), and it is believed that the presence of hope in caregivers can directly impact the sense of hope for those who are ill, suggesting that maintaining hope in family members and caregivers can additionally maintain hope for those who are ill.

This leads to the question of how health professionals can aid in maintaining hope in those who are caring for a person with a terminal illness.

Hope for caregivers in the study by Herth (1993) was defined as "continually unfolding and changing in response to life situations" and as a "dynamic inner power that enables transcendence of the present situation and fosters a positive new awareness of being". In his study of 25 family caregivers, he identified "hope-fostering" strategies to include sustaining relationships, cognitive reframing, time refocusing, attainable expectations, spiritual beliefs, and uplifting energy. Cognitive reframing involved developing a positive outlook on a threatening situation, time refocusing referred to taking a more day-by-day attitude rather than looking too much to the future, attainable expectations described setting attainable goals and being able to redefine their expectations, and uplifting energy referred to learning to balance available energy. He also described threats to maintaining hope, which included isolation, concurrent losses, and poorly controlled symptoms. His results can suggest possible implications for practice, in that efforts should and could be made to aiding those hope-fostering aspects whilst preventing those aspects that are threatening to hope.

It is believed that health professionals such as doctors and nurses can help maintain hope in those who have a terminal illness by "listening carefully to family members, answering their questions, talking with them, and providing useful information" (Duhamel and Dupuis 2003). Treating patients with respect and demonstrating true interest in their physical, psychological, spiritual and emotional health is thought to be a major aspect of bringing comfort and hope to terminally ill patients and their family (Duhamel and Dupuis 2003; Post-White et al. 1996).

In a study of 61 family members of people with terminal cancer, Chapman and Pepler (1998) found that those family members who lacked hope were more likely to experience somatic distress, loss of control, and social isolation. Based on their results they suggest that health professionals (they specify nurses in particular) should be more aware of family members' somatic concerns. They further suggest that "a way of fostering hope, and ultimately health, is to address expressed feelings of anticipatory grief and facilitate coping. Once the grief responses are dealt with, the level of hope would be expected to increase, providing an incentive for constructive coping with loss."

5.6   Role of Spirituality

"Hope has been described as being closely related to spiritual well-being in terms of providing a sense of meaning and purpose to life" (Chaplin and McIntyre 2001).

In light of the above statement, and taking into account the important role of spirituality within maintaining hope in those who are terminally ill (Duhamel and Dupuis 2003; Murray et al. 2004), it seems only fitting that we should consider in more detail this aspect of palliative care within the context of this chapter on maintaining hope.

The definition of spirituality has received possibly as much debate as that of hope, and it will be impossible for us to attempt to discuss in detail the issues involved in its definition, this may be found elsewhere (Hermann 2001; Walter 1997; Wright 2001). Although often spirituality may be linked to religion and God, a more current view is that spirituality can encompass much more than this alone. Puchalski and Romer (2000) describe spirituality as that:

"...which allows a person to experience transcendent meaning in life. This is often expressed as a relationship with God, but it can also be about nature, art, music, family, or community—whatever beliefs and values give a person a sense of meaning and purpose in life".

Spirituality is an important aspect for individuals, and possibly even more so for those who are facing a life-threatening illness (Breitbart 2002; Greisinger et al. 1997). A study by Murray et al. (2004) exploring the spiritual needs of people dying of lung cancer or heart failure and their carers found that spiritual issues were of great importance to both parties in the last year of life. Furthermore, a study by Moadel et al. (1999) of existential needs among 248 cancer patients found that 42% wanted help in finding hope, 40% in finding meaning in life, and 39% in finding spiritual resources. This finding emphasises that spiritual needs among patients do exist.

As in the previous section where benefits of maintaining hope were addressed, there are also benefits that have been shown in having a sense of spirituality. It has been suggested that spirituality or having a religious belief can have a range of benefits including psychological, physiological as well as beneficial effects on quality of life (Brady et al. 1999; Jenkins and Pargament 1995; Koenig 2000; McClain et al. 2003; McIllmurray et al. 2003; Murray et al. 2004; Speck et al. 2004; Stewart et al. 1999). Having a strong sense of spirituality or religion has also been identified as an important aspect of coping with a life-threatening illness (Feher and Maly 1999; McClain, et al. 2003; Speck et al. 2004); with a decreased desire to hasten death (Breitbart et al. 2000; McClain et al. 2003); and also for the relatives of those with a terminal illness, it has been associated with more effective dealing with grief (Walsh et al. 2002).

McIllmurray et al. (2003) in fact suggest that finding out about a patient's spirituality can help "service providers" in predicting needs of patients. They believe this because in their study of 354 individuals they found that those who reported that they had a religious faith were less

likely to need help with such things as information, feelings of guilt, and sexuality, for example. Some have referred to "spiritual suffering" that may be the cause of additional physical or "psychologic" problems in those with a terminal illness (Rousseau 2003), again emphasising the need to address spiritual issues within end-of-life care. Although much research, such as those studies mentioned above, describe an important benefit of having a sense of spirituality among patients, a review by Sloan et al. in 1999 emphasises that it is important to note that some of the literature regarding the benefits of spirituality to the patient may be inconsistent.

Although the need for spiritual care has been recognised in the literature and within palliative care policy and research (Breitbart 2002), it appears that in practice it is largely overlooked, avoided, or that there is some sense of uncertainty as to with whom the responsibility of addressing spiritual needs lies (Murray et al. 2004; Rousseau 2003; Walter 1997). Rousseau in 2000 stated that in fact "physicians rarely inquire about spiritual concerns". Reasons why spiritual needs may not be addressed by healthcare professionals adequately have included a lack of time, inadequate training, lack of confidence in dealing with and understanding of spirituality, uncertainty as to whose role it was to deal with such issues, and feelings of personal vulnerability (Kristeller et al. 1999; Murray et al. 2004). For example, with regard to role uncertainty, Kristeller et al. (1999) found that although many oncologists and nurses identified themselves as responsible for addressing spiritual distress, 85% of these healthcare providers also felt that ideally the role should lie with a chaplain.

Although health professionals avoid addressing spiritual issues, individuals themselves found it difficult to raise issues about spirituality with their healthcare providers in the first place (Murray et al. 2004).

What needs to be considered therefore is what health professionals can do to improve or integrate spiritual care/consideration as part of effective communicating and care with/of patients with terminal illness and their families. Currently there seems to be little guidance in this area, but below are some suggestions found in the literature. Koenig (2000) suggests that it will be important for health professionals to "acknowledge and respect the spiritual lives of patients"; Puchalski and Romer (2000) have suggested that clinicians should include a spiritual history in their consultations in order to help patients with regards to their specific needs, and give guidance on how to take such spiritual histories.

From patients' perspectives, Murray et al. (2004) have identified help in maintaining relationships with families, feeling connected to others and to society, and in participating with church and prayer as ways in which patients can be helped in addressing their spiritual needs. And although they recognise that patients and families do not find it easy to raise issues regarding spirituality, healthcare professionals may be able to help in this by allowing for time, listening, empathy and open questioning. Mathews et al. (1998) suggest that clinicians should ask patients who responded positively to questions about religion and faith what they could do to support them in maintaining their sense of spirituality. There have been some interventions that have directly targeted spiritual well-being (Greenstein and Breitbart 2000); however, the success of such interventions is yet to be clarified (McClain et al. 2003). For further information regarding interventions in this area, please see elsewhere (Breitbart 2002).

As spirituality may be closely linked to hope, and both are important aspects of communication, it is important to consider all these aspects when communicating with individuals. Although there may not be a clear rule or set of guidelines to follow on how best to do this, there is throughout a great emphasis on the importance of providing care that is person-centred and individualised. Creating a comfortable, willing and open environment for discussion and questioning, in conjunction to allowing adequate time and practicing good listening skills and being empathetic, may be the best summary of how to proceed. Allowing for such conditions may facilitate patients in informing the healthcare providers of the needs that are specific to them, which is likely to be beneficial to all aspects of health: physical, psychological, social and spiritual.

5.7   Conclusions

From the wealth of literature available it appears important to express a note of hope when communicating information, news or healthcare plans to patients with cancer, or in fact any serious illness. Whereas in previous years withholding information to protect patients, and the belief that this would not diminish hope, was common practice, more recently truth telling has become the norm. Healthcare staff who are able to empathise and care—as well as providing hope, trust, interest and commitment—are important to patients and their families. This implies that two dimensions of hope should be considered: (a) "patient/family orientations to hope", which involves needing to believe in a miracle and living parallel realities—that is, hoping for a cure or remission whilst at the same time realising the terminal nature of the illness; and (b) "messages from the healthcare providers supporting hope" by using words and approaches that leave the door open, retain professional honesty and respect alternative paths. It is the duty of those health professionals concerned to do what they can to help maintain hope, to promote holistic care, and to maximise physical, social, psychological, and spiritual health, in the true nature of cancer care.

Going Without Saying, by Bernard O'Donoghue

It is a great pity we don't know
When the dead are going to die
So that, over the last companionable
Drink, we could tell them
How much we liked them.
Happy the man who, dying, can
Place his hand on his heart and say:
"At least I didn't neglect to tell
The thrush how beautifully she sings."

References

1. Addington-Hall J, Lay M, Altmann D, McCarthy M (1995) Symptom control, communication with health professionals, and hospital care of stroke patients in the last year of life as reported by surviving family, friends, and officials. Stroke 26:2242–2248
2. Back AL, Arnold RM, Quill TE (2003) Hope for the best, and prepare for the worst. Ann Intern Med 138:439–443
3. Benzein E, Saveman BI (1998) Nurses' perception of hope in patients with cancer: a palliative care perspective. Cancer Nurs 21:10–16
4. Bolmsjo I, Hermeren G (1998) Challenging assumptions in end-of-life situations. Palliat Med 12:451–456
5. Bottorff JL, Gogag M, Engelberg-Lotzkar M (1995) Comforting: exploring the work of cancer nurses. J Adv Nurs 22:1077–1084
6. Brady MJ, Peterman AH, Fitchett G, Mo M, Cella D (1999) A case for including spirituality in quality of life measurement in oncology. Psychooncology 8:417–428
7. Breitbart W (1995) Identifying patients at risk for, and treatment of major psychiatric complications of cancer [review]. Support Care Cancer, 3:45–60
8. Breitbart W (2002) Spirituality and meaning in supportive care: spirituality- and meaning-centered group psychotherapy interventions in advanced cancer. Support Care Cancer 10:272–280
9. Breitbart W, Rosenfeld B, Pessin H, Kaim M, Funesti-Esch J, Galietta M, Nelson CJ, Brescia R (2000) Depression, hopelessness, and desire for hastened death in terminally ill patients with cancer. JAMA 284:2907–2911
10. Bruera E, Neumann CM, Mazzocato C, Stiefel F, Sala R (2000) Attitudes and beliefs of palliative care physicians regarding communication with terminally ill cancer patients. Palliat Med 14:287–298
11. Cantwell BM, Ramirez AJ (1997) Doctor-patient communication: a study of junior house officers. Med Educ 31:17–21
12. Chaplin J, McIntyre R (2001) Hope: an exploration of selected literature. In: Kinghorn S, Gamlin R (eds) Palliative nursing: bringing comfort and hope. Bailliere Tindall, Edinburgh, pp 117–127
13. Chapman KJ, Pepler C (1998) Coping, hope, and anticipatory grief in family members in palliative home care. Cancer Nurs 21:226–234
14. Cutcliffe JR (1995) How do nurses inspire and instil hope in terminally ill HIV patients?. J Adv Nurs 22:888–895
15. Cutcliffe JR, Herth K (2002) The concept of hope in nursing 1: its origins, background and nature. Br J Nurs 11:832–840
16. Dufault K, Martocchio BC (1985) Symposium on compassionate care and the dying experience. Hope: its spheres and dimensions. Nurs Clin North Am 20:379–391
17. Duhamel F, Dupuis F (2003) Families in palliative care: exploring family and health-care professionals' beliefs. Int J Palliat Nurs 9:113–119
18. Edmonds P, Rogers A (2003) 'If only someone had told me . . .' A review of the care of patients dying in hospital. Clin Med 3:149–152
19. Fallowfield L (1993) Giving sad and bad news. Lancet 341:476–478
20. Fallowfield L (1997) Truth sometimes hurts but deceit hurts more. Ann NY Acad Sci 809:525–536
21. Fallowfield L, Ratcliffe D, Jenkins V, Saul J (2001) Psychiatric morbidity and its recognition by doctors in patients with cancer. Br J Cancer 84:1011–1015
22. Fallowfield LJ, Jenkins VA, Beveridge HA (2002) Truth may hurt but deceit hurts more: communication in palliative care. Palliat Med 16:297–303
23. Fanslow CA (1981) The Renaissance nurse. In: Kriger D (ed) Foundations for holistic health nursing practices. Harper and Row, New York, pp 249–272
24. Farran CJ, Keane-Hagerty E, Salloway S, Kupferer S, Wilken C S (1991) Finding meaning: an alternative paradigm for Alzheimer's disease family caregivers. Gerontologist 31:483–489
25. Faulkner A, Argent J, Jones A, O'Keeffe C (1995) Improving the skills of doctors in giving distressing information. Med Educ 29:303–307
26. Feher S, Maly RC (1999) Coping with breast cancer in later life: the role of religious faith. Psychooncology 8:408–416
27. Field D, Copp G (1999) Communication and awareness about dying in the 1990s. Palliat Med 13:459–468
28. Flemming K (1997) The meaning of hope to palliative care cancer patients. Int J Palliat Nurs 3:14–18
29. Ford S, Fallowfield L, Lewis S (1996) Doctor-patient interactions in oncology. Soc Sci Med 42:1511–1519

30. Friedrichsen MJ, Strang PM, Carlsson ME (2000) Breaking bad news in the transition from curative to palliative cancer care--patient's view of the doctor giving the information. Support Care Cancer 8:472–478

31. Girgis A, Sanson-Fisher RW (1998) Breaking bad news. 1: Current best advice for clinicians. Behav Med 24:53–59

32. Greenstein M, Breitbart W (2000) Cancer and the experience of meaning: a group psychotherapy program for people with cancer. Am. J. Psychother 54:486–500

33. Greenwood J (2002) Employing a range of methods to meet patient information needs. Prof Nurse 18:233–236

34. Greisinger AJ, Lorimor RJ, Aday LA, Winn RJ, Baile WF (1997) Terminally ill cancer patients. Their most important concerns. Cancer Pract 5:147–154

35. Hall BA (1990) The struggle of the diagnosed terminally ill person to maintain hope. Nurs Sci Q 3:177–184

36. Hermann CP (2001) Spiritual needs of dying patients: a qualitative study. Oncol Nurs Forum 28:67–72

37. Herth K (1990) Fostering hope in terminally-ill people. J Adv Nurs 15:1250–1259

38. Herth K (1993) Hope in the family caregiver of terminally ill people. J Adv Nurs 18:538–548

39. Herth KA, Cutcliffe JR (2002) The concept of hope in nursing 3: hope and palliative care nursing. Br J Nurs 11:977–983

40. Hickey M (1990) What are the needs of families of critically ill patients? A review of the literature since 1976. Heart Lung 19:401–415

41. Hockley J (1993) The concept of hope and the will to live. Palliat Med 7:181–186

42. Hopwood P, Stephens RJ (2000) Depression in patients with lung cancer: prevalence and risk factors derived from quality-of-life data. J Clin Oncol 18:893–903

43. Hotopf M, Chidgey J, Addington-Hall J, Ly KL (2002) Depression in advanced disease: a systematic review Part 1. Prevalence and case finding. Palliat Med 16:81–97

44. Husebo S (1998) Is there hope, doctor?. J Palliat Care 14:43–48

45. Jenkins R, Pargament K (1995) Religion and spirituality as resources for coping with cancer. J Psychosoc Oncol 13:51–74

46. Kirk P, Kirk I, Kristjanson LJ (2004) What do patients receiving palliative care for cancer and their families want to be told? A Canadian and Australian qualitative study. BMJ 328:1343

47. Kissane DW, McKenzie DP, Bloch S (1997) Family coping and bereavement outcome. Palliat Med 11::191–201

48. Koenig HG (2000) MSJAMA: religion, spirituality, and medicine: application to clinical practice. JAMA 284:1708

49. Koopmeiners L, Post-White J, Gutknecht S, Ceronsky C, Nickelson K, Drew D, Mackey KW, Kreitzer MJ (1997) How healthcare professionals contribute to hope in patients with cancer. Oncol Nurs Forum 24:1507–1513

50. Kristeller JL, Zumbrun CS, Schilling RF (1999) 'I would if I could': how oncologists and oncology nurses address spiritual distress in cancer patients. Psychooncology 8:451–458

51. Kruijver IP, Kerkstra A, Bensing JM, van de Wiel HB (2000) Nurse-patient communication in cancer care. A review of the literature. Cancer Nurs 23:20–31

52. Kutner JS, Steiner JF, Corbett KK, Jahnigen DW, Barton PL (1999) Information needs in terminal illness. Soc Sci Med 48:1341–1352

53. Lo B, Snyder L (1999) Care at the end of life: guiding practice where there are no easy answers. Ann Intern Med 130:772–774

54. Lynch WF (1965) Images of hope. Helicon, Baltimore

55. Matthews DA, McCullough ME, Larson DB, Koenig HG, Swyers JP, Milano MG (1998) Religious commitment and health status: a review of the research and implications for family medicine. Arch Fam Med 7:118–124

56. McClain CS, Rosenfeld B, Breitbart W (2003) Effect of spiritual well-being on end-of-life despair in terminally-ill cancer patients. Lancet 361:1603–1607

57. McIllmurray MB, Francis B, Harman JC, Morris SM, Soothill K, Thomas C (2003) Psychosocial needs in cancer patients related to religious belief. Palliat Med 17:1, 49–54

58. McIntyre R, Chaplin J (2001) Hope: the heart of palliative care. In: Kinghorn S, Gamlin R (eds) Palliative nursing: bringing comfort and hope. Bailliere Tindall, Edinburgh, pp 129–145

59. Moadel A, Morgan C, Fatone A, Grennan J, Carter J, Laruffa G, Skummy A, Dutcher J (1999) Seeking meaning and hope: self-reported spiritual and existential needs among an ethnically-diverse cancer patient population. Psychooncology 8:378–385

60. Moody R (2003) Overcoming barriers to delivering information to cancer patients [review]. Br J Nurs 12:1281–1287

61. Morales E (1994) Meaning of touch to hospitalized Puerto Ricans with cancer. Cancer Nurs 17:464–469

62. Morton R (1996) Breaking bad news to patients with cancer. Prof Nurse 11:669–671

63. Murray SA, Kendall M, Boyd K, Worth A, Benton TF (2004) Exploring the spiritual needs of people dying of lung cancer or heart failure: a prospective qualitative interview study of patients and their carers. Palliat Med 18:39–45

64. Nekolaichuk CL, Bruera E (1998) On the nature of hope in palliative care. J Palliat Care 14:36–42

65. Ong LM, de Haes JC, Hoos AM, Lammes FB (1995) Doctor-patient communication: a review of the literature. Soc Sci Med 40:903–918

66. Owen DC (1989) Nurses' perspectives on the meaning of hope in patients with cancer: a qualitative study. Oncol Nurs Forum 16:75–79

67. Penson J (2000) A hope is not a promise: fostering hope within palliative care. Int J Palliat Nurs 6:94–98

68. Pitceathly C, Maguire P (2003) The psychological impact of cancer on patients' partners and other key relatives: a review. Eur J Cancer 39:1517–1524

69. Post-White J, Ceronsky C, Kreitzer MJ, Nickelson K, Drew D, Mackey KW, Koopmeiners L, Gutknecht S (1996) Hope, spirituality, sense of coherence, and quality of life in patients with cancer. Oncol Nurs Forum 23:1571–1979

70. Puchalski C, Romer AL (2000) Taking a spiritual history allows clinicians to understand patients more fully. J Palliat Med 3, 1, 129–137

71. Quirt CF, Mackillop WJ, Ginsburg AD, Sheldon L, Brundage M, DixonP, Ginsburg L (1997) Do doctors know when their patients don't? A survey of doctor-patient communication in lung cancer. Lung Cancer 18:1–20

72. Rabkin JG, Williams JB, Neugebauer R, Remien RH, Goetz R (1990) Maintenance of hope in HIV-spectrum homosexual men. Am J Psychiatry 147:1322–1326

73. Raudonis BM (1993) The meaning and impact of empathic relationships in hospice nursing. Cancer Nurs 16:304–309

74. Robbins JA, Bertakis KD, Helms LJ, Azari R, Callahan EJ, Creten DA (1993) The influence of physician practice behaviors on patient satisfaction. Fam Med 25:17–20

75. Rogers AE, Addington-Hall JM, Abery AJ, McCoy AS, Bulpitt C, Coats AJ, Gibbs JS (2000) Knowledge and communication difficulties for patients with chronic heart failure: qualitative study. BMJ 321:605–607

76. Rousseau P (2003) Spirituality and the dying patient. J Clin Oncol 21[Suppl]:54–56

77. Sapir R, Catane R, Kaufman B, Isacson R, Segal A, Wein S, Cherny NI (2000) Cancer patient expectations of and communication with oncologists and oncology nurses: the experience of an integrated oncology and palliative care service. Support Care Cancer 8:458–463

78. Siegel K, Raveis VH, Houts P, Mor V (1991) Caregiver burden and unmet patient needs. Cancer 68:1131–1140

79. Silani V, Borasio GD (1999) Honesty and hope: announcement of diagnosis in ALS. Neurology 53 [Suppl 5]:S37–S39

80. Sloan RP, Bagiella E, Powell T (1999) Religion, spirituality, and medicine. Lancet 353:664–667

81. Speck P, Higginson I, Addington-Hall J (2004) Spiritual needs in health care. BMJ 329:123–124

82. Stephenson C (1991) The concept of hope revisited for nursing. J Adv Nurs 16:1456–1461

83. Stewart AL, Teno J, Patrick DL, Lynn J (1999) The concept of quality of life of dying persons in the context of health care. J Pain Symptom Manage 17:93–108

84. Stewart MA (1995) Effective physician-patient communication and health outcomes: a review. CMAJ 152:1423–1433

85. Walsh K, King M, Jones L, Tookman A, Blizard R (2002) Spiritual beliefs may affect outcome of bereavement: prospective study. BMJ 324:1551

86. Walter T (1997) The ideology and organization of spiritual care: three approaches. Palliat Med 11:21–30

87. Wilkinson K (1996) The concept of hope in life-threatening illness. Prof Nurse 11:659–661

88. Wilkinson S, Roberts A, Aldridge J (1998) Nurse-patient communication in palliative care: an evaluation of a communication skills programme. Palliat Med 12:13–22

89. Wright MC (2001) Spirituality: a developing concept within palliative care? Prog Palliat Care 9:143–148

6 Patients and Their Families

P. Firth

Recent Results in Cancer Research, Vol. 168
© Springer-Verlag Berlin Heidelberg 2006

Summary

The focus of this chapter is on how clinicians can understand and communicate with the families of patients suffering from cancer. Most doctors and nurses do not have training in this area and are uncomfortable when conducting interviews with whole families. The need to extend our skills in the family context reflects the changes in the way care is provided to patients with a serious illness. We recognise the part families play in providing care and the subsequent effects on family life. The influence of systemic thinking and social construction theories has led to the acknowledgement that we are all part of systems which interact with each other and it is no longer appropriate to see the patient in isolation. The chapter will look at ideas from family therapy which can help us assess and intervene when necessary.

The patient suffering from a life-threatening illness such as cancer looks to his family and friends for care and support. The management and course of the illness is affected by the involvement of the family and how they manage the stress and the effects of illness on a family member (Wright and Leahey 2000). Duhamel and Dupuis (2003) point out that there are three important factors in the management of the illness: the effects of family stress, the needs of the family as caregivers, and the effects of the role and how the family cope with the way the patient experiences his illness. This presents professionals working in the field with challenges they are often ill-equipped to deal with. Most healthcare workers have inadequate training in understanding family dynamics and even less knowledge about how to communicate effectively with whole families. Consequently, many healthcare professionals avoid couple and family interviews, feeling inadequate and helpless like the families themselves. I will address some of these issues in the chapter, firstly by examining what we now regard as the family and then by using ideas from systemic theory I will look at assessing families, the organisation of families and belief systems, concluding with communications which can bring about change in families needing our help.

Families are complex, they have histories and are influenced by the past. Relationships within families have different meanings and significance not understood unless questions that we ask bring access to them; moreover, their journeys through the illness of the family member is different from that of the patients. However, the need for support/information/valuing/respect is the same. If we are to help, we need to know how to approach families, how to asses their needs, and learn about interventions that help so that we can offer holistic care which will ease the practical, physical, emotional, social and spiritual pain and suffering of the people who will go on living with the significance of the death.

6.1 What Is a Family?

Families are unique, but we can see trends and changes in traditional families. It has been long accepted that the family is the primary group into which we are born and are dependent on for nurturing and socialisation (Altschuler 2005), and we now recognise that families exist within a cultural and social context. Clearly we see great variation in the way people live together, and families will always reflect ideologies which exist in society at any given time (Dallos and Draper 2000).

Family forms have changed due to the influence of divorce, new forms of co-habitation, reconstituted families and the effects of immigration bringing new customs. In the UK, grandparents are increasingly providing childcare as women return to work at a much earlier point in their child's life compared with 20 years ago. Advances in medical science mean that people are living longer and four-generational families are more common.

The salient point to remember is that even if we do not remain in physical contact with our birth families, the connections with them continue to influence our lives. Indeed, researchers in childhood bereavement (Silverman and Nickman 1996) make the point that after a death the relationship with the deceased continues.

6.2 What Happens When a Family Member Has a Life-Threatening Illness?

Adaptation to a close family member having a life-threatening illness requires radical reorganisation of individual and family life (Altschuler 2005). In family life, we make adjustments all the time as children grow and develop and parents age. However, adjustments to the anticipated death of a family member require all the family to reassess their relationship with the ill member and to think about their future. There will be practical arrangements to be made that can have ramifications for child care, for work, finances and social life. Family members become increasingly involved in providing care and managing their own and others' distress (Kissane 2002).

The family life-cycle tasks identified by Carter and McGoldrick (1989) give a perspective of the family as a system moving through time, and focusing on the tasks for each stage. Indeed the death of a close family member is a life-cycle event but sometimes it occurs at what is considered to be the wrong time in the life cycle. The

model helps us to understand the difficulties when a life-threatening illness occurs at a time in the life cycle when the family has other pre-occupations and tasks. An example would be the young family bringing up small children having to cope with the severe illness of one parent or child. Parents with dependent children are put under great strain attending hospital appointments and continuing to care for their children.

Transitional points such as marriage, birth, and adolescence in family life can produce problems of adjustment. The family structure needs to be able to change, e.g. in the case of birth, a couple has to be able to manage being a three-person system. At these transitional points, any family member stress due to serious illness can lead to overload. Understanding family structure in this way helps us to target our help and include all the family. Generally, healthy families negotiate transitional points and maintain family continuity whilst restructuring takes place. However, the threatened exit of a family member has more significance when it occurs at a transitional point. In all our transitions we look at our own histories to guide us. For many families facing a loss the family legacy of loss can be disabling (McGoldrick 1991).

Margaret was 45 years old when she discovered she had breast cancer, her son was 11 years old and her daughter was 7 years old. Margaret was devastated and so was her husband. They had both had significant losses in childhood. Margaret's mother died when she was 3 and she was then cared for by nannies until her father remarried when she was 7 years old. She hated her stepmother and remembers being told or believed that she had caused her own mother's breast cancer which had been diagnosed just after her birth. In her adult life she had very little contact with her father and stepmother. Margaret's husband had been cared for throughout his childhood by a very disabled mother and he married hoping to have a life that was much more unrestricted by illness. The marriage was plunged into difficulty when Margaret became ill and the husband reacted by working longer hours. Margaret had her treatment and was supported by friends who understood her anger. When the cancer returned 2 years later there were fewer friends to help and Margaret came to the attention of the local hospice team where the nurses found her awkward and difficult. Several nurses found them-

selves complained about and the specialist social worker was asked to help.

Margaret needed time to tell her story; in the meantime her widowed stepmother became ill and with the support of her therapist Margaret visited her stepmother several times. Her stepmother had been a friend of Margaret's mother and was able to share some insights about her. Margaret read correspondence she never knew about, thus getting in touch with her own relationship with her mother. The anger began to subside and Margaret joined a therapy group (Firth 2003), lived for several more years and was able to mother her children into adulthood. The husband refused individual help but did occasionally meet with Margaret and her therapist.

Some families find enormous strengths within their family and friendship networks. However, many seriously ill people are lonely despite having families and they feel that it is their duty to die quickly (Craib 1999). The patient may gradually withdraw from life in preparation for death, as we shall see from some case examples, but family and professional carers may also distance themselves from the patient. This attempt to lessen the pain can lead to what some writers describe as social death (Mulkay 1993).

The loneliness of family carers and the effects on their health and the long-term consequences of caring have begun to attract more research and study with the aim to help healthcare professionals consider their interactions with family carers and focus on more appropriate support for carers (Smith 2004).

6.3   Assessing Families

There are many families that do not want help from professionals and use their own resources to manage the situations. However, service user involvement in the planning and delivery of palliative care services encourages us to be creative and flexible for those that do. We must make sure that we are addressing the needs of all family members; for example, it is only recently that palliative care professionals have recognised the importance of involving children. It is vital that we develop assessment tools which will highlight issues that may need intervention even if it is at a later stage. Many people will come back and take

up offers of help providing we are approachable. We need to see assessment as a cycle of assessment, intervention, review (Oliviere et al. 1998).

Where families do need professional help, we are looking at the illness of the patient, what it means to the individual and the family, where the family are in the family life cycle, what resources are available to the family within their social networks and how family belief systems affect the family and the history of the family.

It is useful to first engage the family in building a family tree, as shown in Fig. 1. The family tree or genogram gives us a diagram of the family usually over three generations. In compiling the family tree, the clinician and family begin to develop a relationship which will be the foundation for further work. Communication skills such as active listening are the basis for compiling the history of the family and the sharing of the worries and concerns which are stirred up by the diagnosis of a life-threatening illness. The family tree can also be useful in helping families talk about the way they coped before the patient became ill. The history of illness and loss is laid out for everybody to see. Sometimes families then perceive patterns which they had not recognised before.

In the family tree diagram in Fig. 1 we can see that this young man's terminal illness is occurring at a time in the life cycle when the tasks for the family are to raise dependent children. Furthermore, there is only one set of grandparents to support the family. This family has also had three close members die within the last few years. When the diagnosis of a cancer, which at that stage was thought to be curable, was disclosed the couple felt immediately that he had been given a death sentence. The family had a family script which said that cancer meant death. The paternal grandmother had died before the young couple had met, which was felt as a big loss.

In any psycho-social assessment, clinicians need to take into account the stressors of family life, such concerns as finances, work, school and worries about other practical issues. Transport issues, child minding and temporary care of the sick person make it hard for families to meet with professionals, except in their own homes.

Service user groups often press for more help with information about disease and treatment regimes, but again stress the huge financial im-

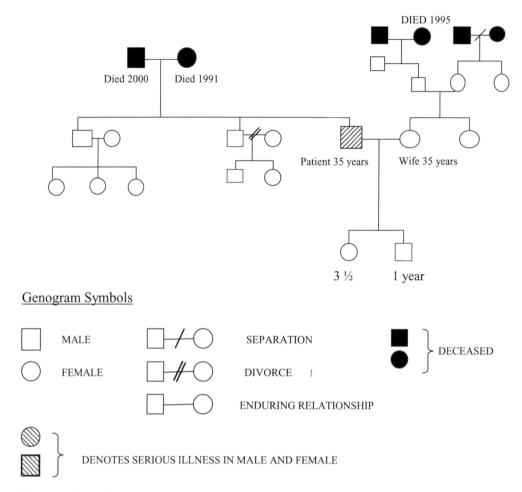

Genogram Symbols

Fig. 6.1 Family tree diagram or genogram

plication of serious illness on the family. We need to ask about this as part of our assessments. Researchers have emphasised the importance of families understanding the process of dying and having an opportunity to express worries (Payne et al 1999). The family will often ask directly for information so that they can plan ahead but can be frustrated and anxious when faced with the uncertainty of prognosis.

One of the most difficult times for patients and families is the change from treatment which is aimed at prolonging life to the terminal stage of the illness. Rolland (1991) identifies this as often ambiguous and urges medical practitioners to make this more explicit so that families can concentrate on the quality of their interactions.

6.4 A Systemic Perspective of Family Life

The conception and early development of family therapy began in the 1950s (Burnham 1999). Therapists began to examine families in terms of the interactions between family members. The individual's symptoms were seen for the first time as being rooted in family patterns of interaction. The family is seen as a system and therefore what happens to one family member has a direct effect on the family as a whole.

Any organisation including families, schools, hospitals, or the local doctor's surgery can be defined as a system (Altschuler 2005). A system is made up of parts which interact with each other and the sum of the parts is different from that of the whole. The importance of balance so that the system is stable, therefore, makes systems susceptible to change. This is sometimes referred to as homeostasis, and indeed there are structures in place to counteract change. Systems always aim to maintain existing patterns of interactions and ways of living.

The value of using a systemic approach is that it focuses our thinking on interactions between family members. Interventions using this approach are designed to strengthen the family's own capacity to resolve issues.

It is generally accepted that a family needs flexibility in managing the demands of a family member having a life-threatening illness. Palliative care practitioners offer a range of supportive care to underpin the family's own coping patterns, but some families may have limited flexibility because of their structure, they may be isolated, living miles from their families of origin (e.g. asylum seekers or refugees) or they may have lost flexibility because they have been caring for a long time. These are families where a family therapy approach may be helpful. Family interventions aimed at helping families are usually brief, focused and, importantly, leave families feeling competent. One example of such an intervention has been recently pioneered in Australia and in the USA: Family-focused grief therapy.

Family-focused grief therapy is a new model of intervention that has been used successfully with families using palliative care facilities (Kissane and Bloch 2002). This therapy relies on screening a family's functioning and identifying those who are at risk of morbid outcome. The importance of the interventions which have been rigorously researched are that they value strengths and identify coping that exist within the family.

I will now address some specific elements from systemic theory which are useful in understanding how families function. These are: open and closed systems, boundaries, belief systems and family scripts.

6.5   Open and Closed Systems

An open system is one in which there is a continuous flow of information from the outside world into the system. This information is reflected on and changes can be made if necessary. This requires the boundaries to be flexible. A closed system uses its rigid boundaries to keep out information that is felt to be threatening to its existence. Ironically, closed systems are more likely to disintegrate because they do not have the creativity to manage changes over time.

Families caring for a family member with a life-threatening disease are faced with a multitude of new threats, not only the likely exit of a family member from the system but also threats from the outside world, as they need to cope with a wide range of health and social care agencies. One 9-year-old boy when asked what was the worst thing about his mother's illness said it was "All the people who had to be in the house each day."

Jenny and her husband had decided to separate when Alan became terminally ill. He had been having an affair with Jane but this finished when Alan became very ill with advanced prostrate cancer. Jenny stayed to look after Alan but was angry and bitter about having to put her life on hold. She saw the nurses who visited Alan as a nuisance and always found fault with them, usually something petty like where they parked the car in the drive. One nurse with the help of a family therapist in the team decided to challenge Jenny, very gently, about what was going on. She said to Jenny that things must be very tough for her and that the nurses felt they were making things worse not better. Jenny responded to this by angrily talking about her situation: Jenny watched the relationships that Alan was making with the nurses, he would be flirtatious and jovial and the final blow for her was that one young nurse was called Jane. Jenny said the nurses coming in each day were a reminder of her husband's infidelity. Alan and Jenny had not spoken about the affair—why it happened and what it meant. Jenny had found out and went immediately to see a lawyer, she was waiting for the finances to be settled when Alan became ill. Jenny and Alan agreed to meet with a therapist for three sessions. In the three sessions the couple were able to reflect on the marriage, their childlessness and the meaning of the affair. Jenny acknowledged her strong obligation to Alan and her anger about this; Alan for his part hated being obligated to Jenny for his care. It was agreed that Alan should go into a hospice for the last few weeks of his life. Jenny visited him regularly and was able to help to arrange Alan's funeral.

This case example shows how a couple were managing an extremely complicated situation involving beliefs about affairs, illness, obligation and the meaning of the illness which they both saw as being a punishment for his affair. It also shows the stress placed on their system by the need to accept healthcare professionals into their system. But finally, opening the system first perceived as a threat became a source for change and adaptation.

6.6 Boundaries

In all systems there is the need for appropriate boundaries. Structural family therapists identify that a confused boundary or no boundaries can lead to stress in the system. An example might be in a family where one parent has a very strong alliance (confused boundaries) with a child and this has the effect of excluding the other parent. Absence of boundaries or confused boundaries are especially problematic when a family member gets ill.

If we consider institutions as systems, sometimes there are no clear boundaries between the management structure and the workforce, which can lead to confusion and workforce stress. In hospices and palliative care units the staff and patients and families get caught up in very powerful dynamics, relationships are intense and the staff members are frequently struggling to manage the boundaries while the patient's body is falling apart. This can be held if the unit has clear structures and tools to support staff and families (Firth 2003).

6.7 Meanings

Meanings which people give to events are important for clinicians if they wish to communicate effectively with families. Systemic theory sug-

gests that meanings which people give to events serve to explain, but they can also restrain us in the actions and choices which we make (Dallos and Draper 2000). Asking a very sick person what they are making of a particular situation will allow us to start where they are, not where we think they should be.

6.8 Belief Systems

An understanding of a family's belief system around the illness of a family member can be very useful in our attempts to offer help. What is a belief system? How does it work and develop?

Mostly the rules which govern our lives in our intimate relationships are not made explicit, although some are. Family therapists suggest that these rules, the way we live our lives, lead to the development of a belief system. It is important to try to understand a family's belief system because it comes into play whenever changes and choices have to be made. Belief systems sustain patterns of behaviour which in turn come from beliefs. Beliefs about the cause of the illness that lead to blame and shame can be particularly difficult in blocking the way a family might work through the knowledge of the illness and become reconciled to the outcome (Rolland 1991).

Wendy and Jo had been married for 20 years. Jo was 15 years older than Wendy and had left his first wife to live with Wendy leaving behind two small children. Jo remained very involved in the lives of his children but they never really accepted Wendy. Jo suffered a great deal of ill health and was eventually diagnosed with terminal lung cancer. Wendy cared for Jo with great devotion but felt that his children did not value or support what she was doing. When Jo was eventually admitted to a specialised palliative care unit, Wendy tried to limit the visiting of Jo's children fearing that she would have to share the last few hours of Jo's life with them. What was behind all this? Wendy's belief was that Jo was not loved by his first wife and children and that she had made his last 20 years very happy. Jo's children believed that Wendy had stolen their father from them—it was deemed to be her fault that their father had left them. The therapist talked to the family together and realised how frightened Wendy and the family were. It was evi-

dent that many of their problems were to do with their early attachments to their parents. Wendy was a young child during the Second World War and suffered significant separations from her parents. Jo's children endured the severe depression of their mother particularly after their father's departure. After recognising that Jo was so important for all of them, they were able to be together for his death.

The case example shows another aspect of belief systems that is important, which is the way things are viewed through these belief systems. They act as a filter that tries to stop things happening which would/could upset the balance of family life. The assumption should never be made that all family members hold exactly the same beliefs about everything. This can be assessed in an interview by checking out with everybody if one belief expressed by one person is confirmed.

We also need to consider our own personal and professional beliefs about serious illness, death and dying. We all have are own belief systems and it is an important part in clinical supervision to examine one's own views, particularly the issue of roles, expectations and professional limits (Fredman 1997).

6.9   Family Scripts

Byng-Hall (1985, 1988) introduced the idea of "family scripts" to describe how family members seemed to repeat patterns of behaviour or scenarios when similar contexts are experienced. He suggested that they act as if they are following a script. The importance of these family scripts means that they can be passed down through generations. This concept can be very helpful when we are trying to understand the behaviour of a family by integration of knowledge from a genogram. One example would be where a family member kills herself whilst suffering from post-natal depression. This creates great anxiety whenever a family member is pregnant and induces a range of protective behaviours leading to a family script around pregnancy which can be passed on through generations unless family members talk about their fears and try to work out different strategies. This idea of families us-

ing models from the past to approach current problems is very common in family therapy. One helpful strategy is to help families find new models.

Creation of rituals is more frequently used in bereavement work but it can also be useful in introducing new ways of approaching difficulties. Some family therapists have noted the lack of rituals in families facing loss (Imber-Black 1988). However, this is not always the case, as the following examples illustrate. One family, for example, always organised to spend an evening together having a take-away meal and a video the week after the mother's chemotherapy. In this way they felt they were celebrating the passing of another treatment.

When Janet's only daughter died suddenly, the problem for her was that she was plunged into echoes from her past. As the first Christmas after her daughter's death approached, her young son and husband desperately wanted to talk about what they were going to do. Janet was locked in her own grief. The family agreed to meet with a therapist. In the session Janet revealed for the first time that she had had an older sister who had died suddenly when Janet was 8 years old. Janet remembers her family being devastated and she called it growing up in the house of death. Her parents never talked about what had happened but took Janet to her sister's grave each week. Her adolescence was lonely and Janet retreated into her books. After university she never returned home to live but married after gaining her degree. Thereafter she did not visit her sister's grave anymore. Janet's husband and son were determined to talk about things and encouraged her to find together her sister's grave. The family visited the grave and from then on gained comfort from the belief that the two girls were in heaven playing together. Although things were very hard the family was determined not to repeat the script of Janet's family, but to talk about their own painful feelings related to loss and grief.

6.10 Tasks and Adjustments for Families with a Terminally Ill Member

It has already been noted that the patient's journey and that of the family is different. The patient has to cope with issues such as pain, fear and increasing dependence. It may be the first time he has been ill, been hospitalised or had an operation. The family members are fearful too but desperately want things to get back to normal. Generally, patients and families treat the first diagnosis as an event that they determine will not change their lives; however, if the disease returns, as with some cancers, they then find it increasingly difficult to maintain this view and this way of functioning. For example, a husband with a sick wife may have to continue working and at the same time to care for his wife and children. Some may have never done this before. Single parents who are ill may have to contact former partners to negotiate long-term child care. All family members face huge uncertainty and often crippling anxiety (Christ 2000), which is new and also puts great strain on family life, making it impossible to continue with life as before.

Increasingly families are reconstituted. The parents may have had several marriages and children live with step-parents. In one family where the mother was very sick the children were told they could not tell their father, who had since remarried. This cut them off from an important source of support. Alliances are complex and old hurts often surface in a time of heightened anxiety. Some elderly patients have lost touch with important relatives because of disputes they cannot even recall. Talking about issues like this can be very rewarding, especially if grandchildren are found and lost sons and daughters are reconciled.

Another major challenge for the family is when the ill person either withdraws or reacts with denial of the illness. Sometimes it is only a matter of time, but for others it can be a major problem.

A young man who had been given a terminal diagnosis refused to accept it. He spent hours on long bike rides with his children. In order to cope with the pain of separation from his family, he withdrew emotionally. *As he got weaker he still dragged himself about the house and refused to talk about his illness with his wife and would only accept minimal pain relief. He did eventually let his family have some support and it became clear that his behaviour was linked to the "silent" death of his own father when he was 7 years old. Sadly he died without being able to say goodbye to his own children thus repeating the pattern of the past.*

A common family issue, particularly when it is an elderly relative who is ill, is "protection". Doctors are often asked not to tell the elderly patient that they are dying so as to spare the patient distress. Should the professionals insist that this should be tackled?

Most healthcare professionals point out that access to services for the seriously ill and dying means those patients have a right to be told the truth about their illness, but some patients then choose to ignore the information.

An elderly man was diagnosed with terminal cancer of the stomach; the surgeon told him he had a tumour but despite this he maintained he had an ulcer. Some family members felt this should be confronted so that he could be involved in planning for his estate. Others felt he would give up if he really faced the truth. In the end, after one family member gently tried to talk to him again about his illness, the family came to the conclusion that this was his way of coping, which had to be respected.

6.11 The Family Interview– Some Common Issues

The problem in inviting families to meet professionals is that sometimes the most important member does not attend; it is therefore important to check this out and concentrate on meeting at convenient times for all. Should the ill person attend? Are you meeting at the family home? The family need to be given some idea about what to expect from the meeting. The clinician must have some idea of what the meeting might achieve. One important task is to build up a relationship with the family so that an alliance is created between the family and clinician. Open questions allow the group to explore important questions and to set an agenda. It is important to first ask about the illness and how it affects each member. Family members should be encouraged to listen and support individuals who are particularly vulnerable. The main objective of the family interview is to enhance the family's own capacity to problem solve.

Some of the most useful sessions involve children. The youngest child will often raise something that other family members might not want to be discussed but which can move things on in terms of support and understanding.

One family was visited a few hours before the mother's death. The father and his three children met with the clinician downstairs whilst the mother was upstairs in bed being attended to by the hospice nurse. The atmosphere was very tense and the 4-year-old boy was playing with toy wrestlers. He kept saying that he could not play because a figure was missing. His sisters knew their mother was dying but he did not. The therapist asked the family what they thought he was talking about. His father then said to his children, "We will manage without mummy, it will be hard but we are a family and will help each other." The 4-year-old stopped playing and climbed onto his father's knee. The other children also hugged their father. The clinician suggested that they could all go together to see the mother upstairs. The children brought in their duvets and slept the night on the floor next to their parents.

Their father understood that his very young children, facing the death of their mother, needed reassurance that their needs would be met (Silverman 2000). This example demonstrates the importance of using techniques which allow families to enhance their capacity to cope with the situation.

This kind of conversation and situation is probably one of the hardest episodes that a parent has to face. We need to respect their decision to tell children about an imminent death or not to tell. However, there is evidence that giving children information appropriate for their age and understanding is helpful and one of the most adequate ways of protecting children (Christ 2000). Generally, as with adults, it is best to approach children by asking them what they think is happening. The clinician must have the trust of the parents to conduct such interviews, during which the parental role and position is always validated.

A social worker met with a mother, father and their two children. Their grandmother, who had advanced breast cancer with brain metastases, was also present. The children were 6 and 4 years old and the adults were concerned that they did not know what was happening. The children had some paper and pens and played on the floor whilst the adults talked about the care of the grandmother, who had come to stay with them. The social worker asked the children to draw their house, which they did, but grandmother was drawn lying down. The children were asked why they had drawn the picture in this way and when they explained that they knew she was very ill. They were given a paper with the outline of a body on it and asked to draw where their grandmother was ill. The children used a red pen to mark the body where the breast was but then used a blue pen to draw three small holes in the head explaining that their grandmother had three bits in her head that made her say silly things. The adults were amazed at the accuracy of the observations. These children showed how much they had communicated with each other without the parents being aware of it.

In the two examples explored, all the parents demonstrated that they were child centred and could think and help the children with their problems. Silverman (2000) examines the differing responses of child-centred and parent-centred families and concludes that after bereavement we need to support parents in providing emotional care which encourages continuity and connection. They need to provide an environment that promotes growth and adaptation which is hard to do when there are so many problems to face.

One of the most effective ways of helping families is to encourage them to tackle things one by one. The aim is to build structures and a sense of competence within the family. It is important for people to feel that they have done the best they can. Each family will develop a story of the illness, what caused it, what it meant and what part they played in the care of their loved one. Sometimes one of the most important functions for supporters of families is to validate "their story" and to help them to gain some understanding, mastery and control over their experiences.

6.12 Conclusions

It is important that the patient and their family are considered when professionals offer care to patients with life-threatening illnesses. Structures and professionals who are competent to provide this care are needed. Concepts from family therapy can help to understand the family as a system and to assess their needs. Meeting the important members of the family can be diagnostic and therapeutic. Increasingly we also need to provide practical support for family caregivers as we move to family situations in which both parents work or the family is a single-parent household.

The importance of relationships which are genuine, respectful, caring and sustaining will help families to manage in the crisis of the terminal illness of a family member. Families tell us of the crippling fear, the waves of anxiety and the rollercoaster of events that they have to endure. We need to do our jobs to the best of our ability, providing medical, nursing, psychosocial and spiritual care alongside practical help and information. Our interventions need to be organised so that we can respond to the changing needs and roles of the patient and the family caregivers as the disease progresses (Perreault et al. 2004).

References

1. Altschuler J (2005) Illness and loss within the family. In: Firth PH, Luff G, Oliviere D (eds) Loss, change and bereavement in palliative care. Open University Press, Maidenhead, pp 53–65
2. Bowlby J (1980) Attachment and loss, vol 3. Loss sadness and depression. Basic Books, New York
3. Burnham J (1999) Family therapy. Routledge, New York
4. Byng-Hall (1985) The family script: a useful bridge between theory and practice. J Fam Therapy, 7:301–305
5. Byng-Hall (1988) Scripts and legends in families and family therapy. Fam Process 27:167–180
6. Carter B, McGoldrick M (1989) The changing family life-cycle: a framework for family therapy, 2nd edn. Allyn & Boston, Boston
7. Christ GH (2000) Healing children's grief. Oxford University Press, Oxford
8. Craib I (1999) Reflections on mourning in the modern world. Int J Palliat Nurs 5::87–89
9. Dallos R, Draper R (2000) An introduction to family therapy. Open University Press, Philadelphia, Buckingham
10. Duhamel F, Dupuis F (2003) Families in palliative care: exploring family and health care professionals beliefs. Int J Palliat Nurs 9:113–119
11. Firth PH (2003) Multi-professional teamwork. In: Monroe B, Oliviere D (eds) Patient participation in palliative care. A voice for the voiceless. Oxford University Press, Oxford
12. Fredman G (1997) Death talk. Conversations with children and families. Karnac Books, London
13. Imber-Black E (1988) Ritual themes in families and family therapy. In: Imber-Black E, Roberts, Whiting R (eds) Rituals in families and family therapy. Norton, New York
14. Kissane D, Bloch S (2002) Family focussed grief therapy Open University Press, Buckingham
15. McGoldrick M (1991) The legacy of loss. In: Walsh F, McGoldrick M (eds) Living beyond loss: death in the family. Norton, New York, pp 104–129
16. Mulkay M (1993) Social death in Britain. In: Clark D (ed) The sociology of death. Blackwell, Oxford
17. Oliviere D, Hargreaves R, Monroe B (1998) Good practices in palliative care. Aldershot Arena Ashgate
18. Payne S, Smith P, Dean S (1999) Identifying the concerns of informal carers in palliative care. Palliat Med13:37–44
19. Perreault A, Fothergill-Bourbonnais F, Fiset V (2004) The experience of family members caring for a loved one. Int J Palliat Nurs 10:133–143
20. Rolland JS. Helping families with anticipatory loss. In: Walsh F, McGoldrick M (eds) Living beyond loss:death in the family. Norton, New York. pp 144–164
21. Silverman PR, Nickman S (1996) Children's construction of their dead parents. In: Klass D, Silverman PR, Nickman S (eds). Continuing bonds: new understanding of grief. Taylor& Francis, Washington, DC, pp 73–86
22. Silverman PR (2000) Children as part of the family drama: an integrated view of childhood bereavement. In: Malkinson R, Shimshon Rubin S, Witztum E (eds) Traumatic and non-traumatic loss and bereavement. Psychosocial Press, Madison

23. Smith P (2004) Working with family care-givers in a palliative care setting. In: Payne S, Seymour J, Ingleton C (eds) Palliative care nursing: principles and practice. Open University Press, Maidenhead, pp 312–328

24. Wright LM, Leahey M (2000) Nurses and families. A guide to family assessment and intervention, 3rd edn. F.A. Davies Company, Philadelphia

7 Children with Cancer

M.A. Grootenhuis, B.F. Last

Recent Results in Cancer Research, Vol. 168
© Springer-Verlag Berlin Heidelberg 2006

Summary

Some specific aspects of communication in pediatric oncology will be outlined in this chapter.
These include openness about the disease, which
has become increasingly important. Furthermore, the law of double protection, a self-protective strategy used by children, parents, and hospital staff, will be sketched out. It is very striking
that protection is often achieved through protection of the other. Several examples of this strategy will be presented. Finally, attention will be
paid to communication about death in the palliative phase.

7.1 Introduction

Today, approximately two-thirds of children
with cancer survive their illness. This means that
one-third of the children diagnosed with cancer
still die as a result of their disease. Survival rates
of children with cancer have increased drasti-
cally over the last decades. In developed countries about 1 in every 1,000 adults reaching the
age of 20 years will be a long-term cancer sur-
vivor. This progress in medical care means that
depending on the course of the illness, the focus
of patient care varies from communicating about
improved survival, treatment protocols for cancer, quality of life of the child and the family, to
communicating about death and palliative care.
Communication in the pediatric setting is essentially different from adult patient care. Not
only the physician and the patient, but also parents participate. Furthermore, physicians have to
deal with emotions of both the children and the
parents, and they have to take the developmental
stage of the child into account.

We will pay attention to three relevant aspects
of communication in pediatric oncology care: (1)
the importance of openness about the disease;
(2) double protection, a self-protective strategy
used by children, parents, and hospital staff, and
(3) communication about death in the palliative
phase. Before these issues are outlined, relevant
information about childhood cancer and functions of communication in pediatric oncology
are described.

7.2 Childhood Cancer

The occurrence of cancer in children is approximately 2% in Western industrialized countries.
Although the incidence of cancer in children is
small, it is still the second leading cause of death
in children and the primary cause of death from
pediatric illness (Smith and Gloeckler Ries 2002).
In The Netherlands approximately 370 children
per year (Visser et al. 1992) are diagnosed with
cancer. Diagnoses typical in childhood cancer
are: leukemias (29%) of which acute lymphocytic
leukemia (ALL) is the most common, namely
22% of all diagnoses; brain and other central
nervous system (CNS) tumors (22%); and cancer
of the lymph glands (Hodgkin and non-Hodg-
kin lymphoma's, 13%). Other malignancies are
less common, such as soft tissue sarcoma (e.g.,
rhabdomyosarcoma 7%), tumors of the kidney
(Wilms' tumor or nephroblastoma, 6%), neuro-
blastoma (6%) or bone tumors (e.g., Ewing and

osteosarcoma, 4%). Besides treatment with chemotherapy, surgery, and radiotherapy, children with cancer are confronted with invasive medical procedures such as bone marrow aspirations, lumbar punctures, and venepunctures. For example, children with ALL face a 2-year treatment protocol with chemotherapy. The treatment starts with the induction phase to induce remission, a state in which the disease is no longer obviously detectable. Further treatment, however, is required to reach cure, and to prevent the occurrence of CNS disease, prophylactic treatment is needed.

7.3 Functions of Communication

Communication established through the exchange of messages between persons has a dual function that is informational and relational. On the one hand, communication has the function of transmitting information to another person. On the other hand, the function is to define, maintain, or alter the relationship with the other person (Penman 1980). The parent who says: "It is time to take your medicine, please don't be a naughty child again" is communicating at an informational level ("it is medicine time") and at a relational level ("be compliant by following my instructions").

In stressful situations the function of communication is of utmost importance. Information increases the controllability of a threatening situation if the child understands what can be done about the situation, how negative consequences can be avoided or ameliorated by his/her own actions. Information thus reduces uncertainty about a threatening situation if it increases the predictability of the situation.

In searching for and developing control, communication about the disease is important for the child and his parents. Communication serves to enhance primary and secondary control and changes the appraisal of the situation and is therefore related to coping. Lazarus and Folkman (1984) define the coping process as:"cognitive and behavioural efforts to manage specific external and/or internal demands that are appraised as taxing or exceeding the re-

sources of a person." One's perceptions, or cognitive appraisals, are important elements in regulating distress or managing the problem causing the distress. Problem-focused coping involves direct efforts to ameliorate the problem causing the distress, whereas emotion-focused coping is directed towards regulating effects surrounding a stressful experience. People not only have emotions, they also handle them, and communication is one of the tools to do so. When a family has to cope with the life-threatening illness of a child, there is little that family members can do to change the situation or exert control over it. Without control, family members have to rely on emotion-focusing coping strategies or cognitive control strategies.

Communication serves for both the primary control of the situation (problem-focused coping) and the secondary control of the situation (emotion-focused coping). Information exchange about the disease and treatment promotes primary control. It enables those involved to define the problem and make attempts to solve it. Communication about the disease directed at secondary control of the situation promotes understanding and acceptance of the disease and aims to reduce negative emotions and strengthen positive emotions. This is illustrated by the parent who maintains telling the child it will get better. With this he or she invites the child to view the situation in a certain (optimistic) way, and thus attempts to reinforce the child's hope and reduce fear.

7.4 Openness About the Disease

For long it was not common to communicate frankly with children about cancer, survival, and death. Fortunately, now it is argued that enabling children to assimilate information and feelings allows them to cope better. Open information to the child with cancer about diagnosis and prognosis has also been found to be beneficial for the child's emotional experience of his situation (Last and van Veldhuizen 1996). In a study about openness of the diagnosis and prognosis, in relation to the emotional well-being of children with cancer, parents were interviewed about the information they had given to their child. Self-report questionnaires were administered to the children measuring anxiety and depression. Children who received open information about their diagnosis and prognosis at the initial stage of the disease showed significantly less anxiety and depression (Last and van Veldhuizen 1996). These findings suggest that parents should be advised to inform their child with cancer openly and soon after the initial diagnosis. Although the perspectives have been improved nowadays in many cases and the message can be given with an outlook on hope and cure, for parents it remains a difficult task to inform the child with cancer about the diagnosis and prognosis (Clarke et al. 2005).

We believe it is important to incorporate openness of information as part of the treatment protocol, obliging hospital staff members to help the child to understand this information and to support the child and parents in their attempts to gain psychological control of the situation. It is important to leave it up to the child how often he or she wants to discuss the illness and his or her emotional experience. The child should not be forced to talk about it, but the often subtle hints which children give should be responded to.

Tension exists between the need to control the situation through protection and the need to share thoughts and emotions with the other person. If the threatening stimuli and the emotions are too strong to be coped with or to be denied, then the need for protection and support increases. On the other hand, open information enables the child to discriminate between imaginary facts and possible implications of facts. By supplying the facts and simultaneously offering reassurance and hope of a favorable outcome, the child will be in a position to build up self-protection. Open information is therefore a necessary condition for effective self-protection.

7.5 Double Protection

In the communication between the child and the parents, it is very striking that protecting oneself is often achieved through protecting the other. Attempts to influence the other person's appraisal in order to reduce the other person's negative emotions not only involve compassion and empathy, but also serve to protect oneself against confrontation with the other person's emotions. This is called the law of double protection. It is essential for the child to believe that his or her parents are strong: if they can handle the situation, it constitutes the signal that the threat can be averted and boosts the confidence that the child will survive. All attempts by parents who conceal the true meaning of the situation from the child are attempts neither to burden nor to weaken the child. The parents' avoidance of discussing their worries and grief related to the illness prevents the child from thinking about it, but also protects the parents from being confronted with the child's emotions.

Not only do parents achieve self-protection through the other person, the child achieves it as well. Not asking questions which might worry the parents, hiding grief, and being brave are attempts of preventing the parents from becoming distressed, and themselves from becoming overwhelmed by the parents' emotions.

The phenomenon of double protection is observable as: (1) parental attribution of positive properties and dispositions to the child and the need of parents to create a positive image of the child; (2) avoidance of communication about the seriousness and the emotional experience of the illness and encouragement to act in a way of mutual pretense; (3) distortion of reality by (partial) denial, the use of symbolic language, and projection of feelings onto other persons. Some illustrations will clarify this.

7.5.1 Illustrations of Double Protection

Positive Attribution We have found support for the hypothesis that parents of children with cancer need to see their children as strong and that they adopt a positive perspective when looking at their children (Grootenhuis et al. 1997). Parents (n=321) and their children (n=205) in different conditions (cancer in remission and with a relapse, asthma, and healthy controls) completed questionnaires to investigate parents' attribution of positive characteristics to their children. It was found that parents of children with cancer attributed significantly more cheerful behavior to their children than parents of children with asthma and parents of healthy children. The findings obtained were equivalent for the mothers and the fathers. We believe that, in order to be able to count their child among the lucky ones who will survive the disease, parents create an image of vitality and zest for life. This positive attribution by parents of children with cancer may be a beneficial coping strategy as long as the emotional feelings of children are not underestimated. Caregivers should be aware of this coping strategy, especially if this coping strategy is out of balance or pathological. It can also be possible that children give their parents the impression they are doing fine to protect their parents from the more negative emotions resulting from the stressful situation.

An example of double protection in a family which was troublesome for the child is as follows. During a research project interviewers were given the impression by parents that their girl was cheerful and optimistic. The parents described their daughter as being unaware of the dangers and consequences of her disease. The impression of the researcher who interviewed the girl, however, contradicted this image. During the interview, the girl told the interviewer that she still worried a lot about her illness and about a possible recurrence. Furthermore, she told the interviewer that she often cried in her room, and she said: "My cuddly toy absorbs all my tears." She said that she did not want to bother her parents with this because they always said that there was no reason to be afraid. The girl had a high score on a depression questionnaire. This example illustrates that the emotional experiences of children with cancer may be ignored if their parents attribute too many positive characteristics to them because they need to see their child as strong. The need to see the child as strong may also become harmful if illness-related symptoms are ignored or underestimated. However, if there is considerable agreement between positive attribution and the emotional experiences of the children, and both the parents and the children are able to fight the experience of childhood cancer by adopting this coping strategy, there is no reason to interfere.

If the parents of children with cancer attribute positive characteristics to their children, this may

have consequences on who clinician or researchers will choose to obtain valid information about the child's health and psychopathology. Caregivers must realize that if they ask parents of children with cancer to report about their children, the parents' perception might be obscured by the use of this coping strategy.

Avoiding Communication Open information about the diagnosis and prognosis is found to be associated with a positive influence on the child's emotional reactions, as we have described before. Although most of the children with cancer are aware of the seriousness of their disease, it is found that the communication about the disease between the child and parents is mainly about the necessity to continue treatment and to undergo painful medical procedures and not about the emotional impact of the situation. Once, a 9-year old boy stated: "During her visits in hospital my mother always cried. Then I had to cry too. Once I said: 'If you don't cry anymore, I wont cry anymore.' From that moment on she never did cry again. She always smiled when she visited me." This statement illustrates the child's attempt not only to block the expression of sadness of his mother, but also the child's implicit proposal of mutual pretense: "Let us act as if we are not sad, let us behave as if there is no reason for crying." The conflict between the need to express feelings of distress and the need to protect oneself against these emotions can be solved by a (partial) distortion of reality. Parents who show their grief in front of their child frequently do not give an explanation or they deny that their child's illness is the cause. Illustrative is a mother who says: "When it happened once, he said: 'Mommy, are you crying?' 'No dear, I have a cold,' I said." Communication about the emotional experience can also take place in a symbolic language. An example of this type of communication is provided by a mother in a discussion group for parents. This mother talks about her 11-year-old son, who talked in his sleep while dreaming. In the morning when she asks which of her children had such a troubled sleep, he initially remains silent. She encourages him: "Was that you? Come on, you can tell your mother everything. Dreams are just lies anyway." Then her son tells her that he had dreamed about a physician who told him that he should be dead for 1 year. In the communication between this mother and her son, the expression of fear of death is embedded in the reassurance that dreams are lies and in the magical conception of a temporary death.

Another example of double protection is found in the phenomenon of projection of feeling onto other persons. It is frequently found that children with cancer can worry about the well-being of their parents. In self-report questionnaires and interviews children agree remarkably often with statements referring to something bad that can happen with the family or their parents. With the expression of feelings of anxiety about their parents, the child probably shows feelings of anxiety about his own vulnerability in a self-protective way, whereas parents onto which anxieties are projected, are protected against worrying for their child.

7.5.2 Double Protection by Pediatric Oncology Staff

Above we described the phenomenon of double protection in pediatric oncology by children and parents, sometimes observable by attributing positive characteristics to one another. In relation to this, we speculate that staff members may also need to see children with cancer and their parents as strong, and presumably achieve self-protection via attributing positive characteristics to children and/or their parents. Staff members have to confront children and parents with bad news, with burdensome treatment regimens, and painful medical interventions. Because of the intensity and length of care involved, a strong emotional relationship usually develops between the patient and staff. During the course of treatment, staff members may be confronted with situations in which they are uncertain about the benefits and risks of their work. It is conceivable that if they create an image of children and parents who are able to manage the situation, it enables them to continue their work and to endure the continuing confrontation with the emotional turmoil of the family. With more years of experience in oncology this need to see children and parents as strong may even become increasingly necessary as a coping strategy.

In a study conducted in our department, a to-tal of 76 staff members, 84 children with cancer, and their 163 parents participated (Grootenhuis et al. 1996). We compared staff members' ratings with the parents' ratings on the need for support and with the children's ratings on experienced pain. We found that both gender and number of years working in oncology care were positively associated with increased self-protective reactions in staff members. Male staff members rated medical procedures and the pain children experience in general as less painful than did female staff members. Their judgments about experienced pain in general and the lumbar puncture procedure in particular tended to be lower than the children's ratings. Female staff members attributed more positive characteristics to children with cancer and their parents than did male staff members. Staff members with more years of experience in oncology tended to rate all three medical procedures as less painful than those with fewer years of experience, and they also attributed more positive characteristics to the children. Although some limitations of the study should be taken into account (small numbers, general ratings), we believe that these data provide some support for the hypothesis that staff members' perception is influenced by so-called 'double protection'.

There is no doubt that pediatric oncology staff members need a certain professional distance to cope with the stress of their work. However, care should meet the needs of the children with cancer and their parents. The staff's tendency to attribute positive qualities to children and parents should not interfere with decisions about administration of pain medication or the referral to other additional support services. For this reason, it would not only be desirable to pay attention to the coping strategies of both children with cancer and their parents during medical education programs, but also to focus on self-protective behavior in staff members themselves.

7.6 Communication During the Palliative Phase

If the disease cannot be cured treatment will be focused on palliation. However, in most cases it is not possible to define the terminal period very clearly. Often, the child with cancer is on a gliding scale with declining chances, by which the pendulum of hope and fear remains present for a long time. In these circumstances an important role is reserved for the physician. Giving open information by telling the child and the parents that the treatment is no longer aimed at curing the disease but at palliation of symptoms will commence the process of grief and mourning. Studies show that children wish to be informed about their illness and plans for treatment (Wolfe et al. 2002).

In communication with children with cancer the question that always arises is what do children understand about their disease, treatment, and about death. This is always dependent on their developmental level. Healthy toddlers consider death as a separation or as sleep, which is reversible. The definite character of death is not yet part of their world. This awareness becomes concrete during the school period. At the age of around 12, children are aware that everybody dies including themselves (Eiser 1990). For children who have cancer the development of this process becomes intensive, being confronted with their own mortality and the awareness that children die as well.

We believe physicians have the responsibility to help parents in bringing the message to the child about the forthcoming death. In breaking the bad news they should pay attention to how parents are going to inform their child. However, also for pediatric oncologists this is difficult (Beale et al. 2005).

In the palliative phase it is important that the child can express his thoughts and emotions about the approaching death. In this period children need to be ensured that they will not stay alone and they will not endure unnecessary pain. The words that will be used to describe what death is about will depend on the family's beliefs, religion, and the age of the child. Some children want to talk specifically about certain wishes, about what they want to do once again or about the organization of the funeral. Young children may discuss these matters in an indirect way, by making a drawing or by telling a story. In the approach of the child it is important to be open for these subtle hints.

For the parents, the message that the child can no longer cured is a shock. Disbelief and the notion that what was feared is becoming reality often go hand in hand at this stage. Thoughts about how the death of their child might come, about the funeral, but also about what fine moments with the child will be missed, evoke feelings of pain and grief. Sometimes parent do not communicate with each other about these thoughts and feelings in order to protect each other.

Often parents fear the way their child will die. Will my child suffer from needless pain? Will it happen when I am not there? In this period parents are often very irritable. They may be angry with the physician who cannot cure their child, but also with persons in their environment, because they are in a condition of heightened irritability with little interest in others who may not be able to follow closely the condition of the diseased child. During the child's illness parents also suffer from feelings of guilt. These feelings might arise from perceived shortcomings in meeting the needs of the child, or from asking the question if everything has been done to cure the disease. In the palliative phase, most parents live in a situation of heightened alertness. Somehow condemned to passivity, they may be very active and want to spend most of the time with the dying child. Sometimes they doubt whether they are strong enough to hold on. Especially if other burdensome circumstances are present like marital conflicts, unemployment, illness in other family members, or financial problems.

Finally, for parents it is of importance to experience moments of warm closeness, of intimacy with the child on which they can look back gratefully later on, and many describe a change of values in their life. Some striving (e.g., material wishes) becomes less important, while others, like enjoying family time, are more valued now. In many cases these changes of values are long lasting.

In conclusion, current therapeutic interventions should aim for a declining child to die without physical pain, fear, or anxiety. This implicates that he or she receives adequate medical, spiritual, and psychological support, and that the child at no point feels abandoned. Palliative care, in the terminal phase of cancer, has to be tailored to the different needs and desires of the child and the family, with the goal of providing the best possible quality of life for the days that remain.

References

1. Beale EA, Baile WF, Aaron J (2005) Silence is not golden: communicating with children dying from cancer. J Clin Oncol 20:3629–3631
2. Clarke SA, Davies H, Jenney M, Glaser A, Eiser C (2005) Parental communication and children's behaviour following diagnosis of childhood leukaemia. Psychooncology 14:274–281
3. Eiser C (1990) Chronic childhood disease. an introduction to psychological theory and research. Cambridge University Press, Cambridge
4. Grootenhuis MA, Van Der Wel M, De Graaf-Nijkerk JH, Last BF (1996) Exploration of a self-protective coping strategy in pediatric oncology staff. Med Pediatr Oncol 27:40–47
5. Grootenhuis MA, Last BF, Van Der Wel M, De Graaf-Nijkerk JH (1997) Parents' attribution of positive characteristics to their children with cancer. Psychol Health 13:67–81
6. Grootenhuis MA, Last BF, De Graaf-Nijkerk JH, Van Der Wel M (1998) The use of alternative treatment in pediatric oncology. Cancer Nurs 21:282–288
7. Last BF, van Veldhuizen AM (1996) Information about diagnosis and prognosis related to anxiety and depression in children with cancer aged 8–16 years. Eur J Cancer 32A:290–294
8. Lazarus RS, Folkman S (1984) Stress, appraisal, and coping. Springer, Heidelberg Berlin New York
9. Penman,RA (1980) Communication processes and relationships. Academic Press, London
10. Smith MA, Gloeckler Ries LA (2002) Childhood cancer: incidence, survival, and mortality. In: Pizzo PA, Poplack D (eds) Principles and practices of pediatric oncology. Lippincott, Williams & Wilkins, Philadelphia, pp 1–12
11. Van Veldhuizen AM, Last BF (1991) Children with cancer: communication and emotions. Swets & Zeitlinger, Amsterdam
12. Visser O, Coebergh JWW, Schouten LJ (1992) Incidence of cancer in the Netherlands. Fourth Report of the Netherlands Cancer Registration
13. Wolfe J, Friebert S, Hilden J (2002) Caring for children with advanced cancer integrating palliative care. Pediatr Clin North Am 49:1043–1062

8 Interdisciplinary Communication

F. Porchet

Recent Results in Cancer Research, Vol. 168
© Springer-Verlag Berlin Heidelberg 2006

Summary

After an introduction clarifying the notion of interdisciplinarity, this chapter focuses on the importance of specific roles and mutual responsibilities within the interdisciplinary team, as well as basic rules of communication respecting the values of the concerned partners and professionals, as well as patient and family. Finally, the communication structure for efficient teamwork, and the importance of building a common vision, sharing leadership and learning to work together will be discussed.

8.1 Introduction

As a registered nurse for more than 30 years, I have had the opportunity to fulfil various functions as a nurse, health counsellor, patients' groups moderator, palliative care educator, coach, supervisor and post-traumatic debriefer. Those functions have led me to meet numerous colleagues from various professional contexts: hospitals, homecare, homes for the elderly and institutions for those with physical and learning disabilities. It is through all those meetings with doctors, nurses, social workers, chaplains, physiotherapists, etc. that my knowledge has increased about the specific skills various other professionals can offer to terminally ill persons and those close to them.

It was also my work as a palliative care educator which aroused my curiosity concerning my own understanding of interdisciplinarity. Referring to the definition of Lassaunière and Plagès [1], the expression "interdisciplinary" defines the dynamic between persons who share together experiences from the perspective of their professional knowledge. It is important not only to weave together such knowledge succinctly, but also to mix them through dialogue so that they become mutually reciprocal, in order that each one's competencies will be enriched and the understanding of the situation improved. Interdisciplinarity is thus a new way of organising hospital work, in direct contrast to the traditional model.

In the health field, it means breaking from the traditional work model, in which each practitioner is only concerned with his specific sphere of practice, immersed in his own preoccupations.

In order to highlight an interface between professions and disciplines, there must be a common core of interest, common values and a shared project between the different actors. Above all, there is a need for each partner involved to be aware that he could be enriched by sharing knowledge and values with other professionals, as long as he shows humility in postulating that the person facing him might be equally competent and that they could learn from one another in each circumstance. As Bolly and Vanhalewyn [2] emphasise, working in an interdisciplinary team means accepting risks and, even before that, facing that one's practice could transform through such sharing with other professionals .

8.2 Sharing a Common Goal: The Quality of Life of the Patient and His Family

"A clinical picture does not only consist of a photograph of a patient in his bed; it is an impressionist painting, with his house, his work, his family, his friends, his joys, his sorrows, his hopes and fears surrounding him." These words, written by Peabody in 1927, cited by Dame Cicely Saunders [3], founder of the modern palliative care movement, clearly underlines that severe illness affects a human being in all his dimensions. When suffering invades daily life, when life falls into uncertainness, the physical, psychological, social and spiritual turmoil generates numerous questions to which the patient and his family try to find answers. This is why the interdisciplinary approach by different members of the team, such as nurses, care attendants, doctors, social workers, physiotherapists, chaplains, psychologists, volunteers and others, is meaningful. This is one of the main guarantees: to care and accompany a severely ill patient and his family and friends in all the dimensions of their suffering; it enables us to take into account the physical aspects—related to illness, symptoms and treatments—as well as psychological, spiritual and social aspects.

The quality of care not only depends on the degree to which the professional is prepared to provide assistance but also on sound specific technical and relational knowledge shared within the team. Let us examine, for example, what it means to take into account not only the pain itself, but the "patient in pain" according to the global pain concept described in the WHO technical report No. 804 [4].

In brief, understanding pain consists of an accumulative knowledge related to different domains: anatomy, physiology, physiopathology, pharmacology, psychology, etc. Indeed this knowledge is essential, but not necessarily sufficient; knowledge should lead to the notion of competence. According to Le Boterf [5], "competence is not an accumulation of knowledge, but

a validated know-how in a complex professional situation with the view of a particular purpose". Specifically in relation to pain, this definition, which seems complex and theoretical, becomes meaningful. The know-how leads to a reflective process followed by actions. It is a matter of (1) observing which manifestations of pain the patient shows (verbalised or not), (2) evaluating, recording and referring concerns to team members, (3) explaining in a comprehensible way to the patient and family which treatment will be commenced and why, (4) obtaining consent and beginning an appropriate treatment, (5) checking its effects through pertinent tools and (6) re-evaluating as necessary. Examining a patient in the context of his total pain, listening attentively to him, sharing questions and doubts within the team, referring him perhaps to pain-management specialists, contacting a chaplain who might help the patient who questions the global meaning of his illness—these actions demonstrate how competence is validated know-how. I say "validated" because the professional is not only self-competent, his technical and relational competence can only be validated through others, i.e. the patient, the patient's family, and team members.

Clearly, addressing pain is a significant example of caring for patients with cancer, but the reality of oncological situations cannot be based solely on the pain symptom, even though it is crucial. The intricacy of multiple symptoms, in addition to the existential crisis, obliges the team members to search for an acceptable balance between advantages and disadvantages of possible treatments, based on the patients wishes. Therefore, there is a need for a process of ethical deliberation, with the main interest and goal of trying to determine the conditions for clinical practice based on respect for severely ill patients. As the SFAP College of Palliative Nursing mentions [6], it is a decision-making process illuminated by the light of interdisciplinarity.

How should a practitioner react when facing a patient who refuses medication, while he, as a professional, knows that the treatment would contribute to improving the patient's quality of life? Which steps should we take when a dying patient would like to return home, even when the high probability of complications from his illness seems to suggest otherwise? Standing back and analyzing a conflict situation between a patient and his family/carer without getting involved in one side or the other. Realizing what can be learned from an experience of care. Daring to be creative in meeting particular demands of patients when it seems unrealistic. Affirming one's personal and professional values through a process of ethical deliberation in order to support the patient's choices. These examples clearly show that taking care of a patient with advanced cancer cannot be the privilege of one professional alone in any circumstances, as competent as he might be. These examples show that taking care of a patient, especially the severely ill, cannot be the privilege of one professional alone, as competent as he might be. Let us take another example of a patient complaining about back pain: The physician will think about a spinal cord compression due to metastases and ask for confirmatory tests, the social worker may notice that the patient only complains when the family visits him and will suggest a family meeting, and the nurse will propose a relaxing bath relieving tension due to the position in bed. The risk of a conflict in the team could be related to the fact that each member of the team thinks that his point of view is the most important without taking in account the other professionals' opinions. Meeting the needs of a patient requires then multiple competences that many caregivers from different professions will have to share in order to offer the best quality of comfort and care. It is a common project in which each team member will inculcate his own competencies. This is the essence of interdisciplinarity.

8.3 Appreciating Specific Roles and Mutual Responsibilities

What exactly has been the position of interdisciplinarity in our hospital systems over the years? I suggest that multidisciplinarity is omnipresent in the current care structures—in that there is a diversity of health professions and a multiplicity of medical specialties—but the same cannot be said concerning interdisciplinarity. Patient-centred practice requires time for reflection in order to articulate one another's competencies in a

complementary instead of in an oppositional or parallel way. This is a common project in which each professional has the possibility, or might have so, to make a specific contribution. For this purpose, one should know his own field of action and be able to communicate it, as well as one has to know of the competence of other team members and be able to appreciate their specific contribution. I remember a clinical situation that I met in a hospital in Paris, about 10 years ago. During a meeting with physicians, nurses, care-attendants, social workers and physiotherapists, the case of a woman, approximately 80 years old, was presented. The patient was suffering from dementia and multi-metastatic bowel cancer; she was complaining of fatigue, was falling repeatedly, but could not commit herself to stay in bed, as she had always been very active. During this meeting, the doctor proposed a blood transfusion, aimed at comfort, in order to let her recover her strength and decrease the risk of falling. After explaining why he was proposing this, he turned to ask each person present for their opinion. The care-attendant, invited to share her views, expressed her doubts about the proposition, making the team aware that every time she was taking care of this patient, during washing and dressing, the patient refused to wear red coloured clothes and began to show signs of anxiety. "Every time she sees her red clothes, she is so scared that she begins to tremble, shaking her whole body. I think that she could be panic-stricken to see the transfusion drip in her arm." She evidently was the only one to have observed those details, which might seem insignificant. Because it was appreciated as a pertinent opinion, her remark was taken in account and the team took the decision with the patient's permission to hide the perfusion-holder and the transfusion with a white bed sheet and set it behind the bed, out of the patient's view. This example shows how each member of the team can hold significant details which can contribute, if they are shared within the team, to the patient's care by giving personalised quality treatments and care.

Having many professionals gravitating around a patient does not guarantee that they will work in an interdisciplinary manner. Interdisciplinarity is time demanding: time for meetings, dialogue and questioning teamwork. Interdisciplinarity can be learned progressively through the mutual efforts of each team member with respect for all. At first, the benefit of working in an interdisciplinary team is inversely proportional to the efforts provided and required. One must learn to understand oneself and to get to know the other professionals. Working in interdisciplinary teams is not synonymous with role overlap, where everyone does everything. Obviously, the roles within the team caring for an advanced cancer patient are not as clear as in an operation room, for example. It might happen that a patient shares his spiritual distress with the nurse during a care episode. It is also possible that a chaplain visiting a patient notices that she is sitting uncomfortably in her armchair and helps her to position herself. However, competences can overlap without erasing the specificities related to each professional, nurse, chaplain or other. It is the attitude of professionals towards each other which determines if "interdisciplinary communication" leads to a patient-centred partnership or power struggles within the team. According to Girardier [7], "medical decisions belong to the physician and are his responsibility. Palliative situations are complex and decisions are difficult. The ethical team's capacities are shaken and generally the choices have to be made with uncertainty. The physician is responsible for his acts, but he needs clarification through active participation of the team before taking decisions. Nurses have never demanded to take medical decisions, they only ask for participating actively in the discussion." Unfortunately experience shows that action is often favoured over reflection, while it would be so crucial to think about fundamental values and interpersonal relations in order to reach a full consensus. It is precisely in these uncertain clinical situations where interdisciplinary team members are pressured by time and institutional constraints that they should step back and take the time to consider together the best possible solution. Reflection is not time-wasting but enhances middle and long-term goal-setting, for the benefit of the patient, caregivers and the team itself.

In clinical situations, each member of the team should identify and differentiate his capabilities in terms of competencies, expectations and actions. Clarifying roles within the team,

defining the functions and responsibility level for each one, explicating the problem solving and decision-taking processes, these are key elements for fruitful interdisciplinary teamwork, as long as they are embraced by all members of the team, graduated or not. This means that the success of interdisciplinary teamwork is not only dependent upon the concerned actors' will but also upon institutional demands. Lassaunière and Plagès have noticed that "the main difficulty consists of being actors in a system where individual success is valued, as well as professional division into sectors, corporatism, hierarchy and separate actions which generate power struggles or dynamics". Pre-graduate education contributes to promote this system. In medical education, the pedagogical methods do not integrate teamwork, and medical and nursing students are scrupulously separated. Often in post-graduate education too, physicians, nurses and care-attendants are trained in separate places, and many doctors still do not like to participate in courses with nurses. Nevertheless doctors, nurses, care-attendants and many others have to work together in daily practice, despite their specific cultures. Working together as an interdisciplinary team does not go without saying. There are many elements inhibiting efficient interdisciplinary collaboration: differences of professional education and culture, prejudices, ignorance of the various competences or lack of clarification concerning roles and responsibilities.

8.4 Communicating in the Respect of Everyone's Values

In order to counterbalance all the potential barriers mentioned above, the indispensable cement to building teamwork consists of communication and dialogue. According to Drilling [8], before anything else, each representative of each profession should look introspectively at his way of functioning by asking himself: Why do I have so much interest in this question? Is my approach to this question the only one possible, and why do I favour it? Which questions am I not able to answer and why? How did I obtain this knowledge and why do I use this method?

Experience shows that often a particular profession's jargon is a hindrance to facilitating communication and mutual understanding due to the idiosyncrasies of language, representation and words. As Saunders reminds us, "there are rules for efficient communication in interdisciplinary meetings. One must learn the appropriate language to communicate. Professional jargon, even with other professionals, is unproductive."

To communicate involves meeting other persons in respect of their differences. It means clarifying one's own needs and expectations as well as inviting the others to express their needs and expectations; it means defining together a common sphere of action, the interface; it means being honest and authentic in the relationship; it means recognising one's own limitations in terms of knowledge, competences and levels of responsibility. Such communicating finally means abandoning the glut of prejudices which spoil the quality of the relationship between collaborators. For example, before young physicians arrive in hospital units, one can often hear the following comments in the nursing teams "... and now we have to adjust to a new doctor ... hopefully he or she will be smarter than the previous one ... another very young one who has all the theory in his head but has never seen a patient ... this means again and again explaining the routine, etc." On the physician side, the comments are different "... when I think that I am only now used to all of the routine of this unit, it seems to me that I began yesterday... three months is just enough to get to know the basics to function correctly and be accepted by the nursing team ... hopefully I will not be again facing a nursing team, making me feel like an incompetent person ...." It is evident that the way of looking at the other professional, even before meeting him, influences the way of considering him. How can one build basic confidence for working in an interdisciplinary team for the benefit of patients with thoughts and comments like these?

8.5 Structuring Communication for Efficient Teamwork

The patient and his family should be the centre of the interdisciplinary team, and the information about how they live through illness and its multiple consequences is essential to plan appropriate care. In this sense, the patient and his family should take part in all decisions, since they are the only ones who can express what is most meaningful at each moment of their illness. Patients are our teachers, but only if we, as team members, are able to listen attentively to them with our minds and our hearts. Handling information concerning a patient within the team needs perceptiveness, tact and sensitivity. Everything that has been said to one caregiver in an authentic and trustful climate does not necessarily need to be shared with the whole team. The profound meanings behind words are to be received as real gifts in a spirit of human fraternity, from human being to human being. On the other hand, there are some situations when the patient asks the caregiver to keep a secret for himself; the caregiver must then be careful not to be trapped in a promise that he will be unable to keep, knowing the potential negative consequences of such a promise. In this situation, one should gently yet succinctly convey to the patient that one understands his demand but that it is crucial to share some information within the team, in order to adapt care and be able to accompany him as adequately as possible at this time of his life. Data concerning the physical, psychological, social and spiritual patient's dimensions enable the team to define the best therapeutic project for the patient and his proxies. Passing information within the team is one of the most essential elements for interdisciplinary communication.

In the hospital, at home or in any other care setting, the "transmission tools" represent adequate structures to support communication between professionals and to provide continuity of care:

Symptom Assessment Tool We will not discuss here the relevance of symptom assessment scales. It is essential, however, to mention how any symptoms assessment tool can represent a cohesive approach within the interdisciplinary team, as long as all the team members use the same tool in the same way. This gives them the opportunity to speak the same language through a common reference code to qualify and quantify the patient's comfort.

Patient's Record The patient's record is another key element for the transmission of data between professionals. If possible, each team member should access it in order to look for information as well as to transcribe care observations or actions. Physiotherapist, social worker, physician, nurse, chaplain, care-attendant or any team member will be more motivated to work within an interdisciplinary spirit if he perceives that his contribution is essential to the realisation of the common goal.

Liaison Book Bolly and Vanhalewyn emphasise the importance of the liaison book, which is a very simple and useful tool allowing not only improvement to interdisciplinary teamwork, but it also acts as a time-saving initiative. Experience shows that the liaison book allows the patient and his caregivers to become active partners in care by giving them the opportunity to write down potentially relevant information for when the nurse or physician or physiotherapist visit.

Telephone The telephone is often used abusively in our care settings, but nevertheless it represents a rapid and performing communication tool, particularly when it is urgent to pass information related to patient's transfer from one care setting to another. How many times did we hear general practitioners complaining that they did not receive any information concerning a patient leaving hospital late on Friday afternoon or that the home nurse was not informed about the patient's return? Conversely, home care or elderly home teams do not pass global information about the patient's habits, his difficulties related to his illness or the worries he might have concerning the treatments, which complicates acute care teamwork.

Team Meeting Frequently we hear in our hospitals that team meetings are time-consuming and one does not understand why so much time should be used for them. But there are basic rules for fruitful team meetings as efficient communication tools. First of all, the objective of the meeting and the importance of one's presence should be known by each member. The meeting's length

should be clearly defined as well as the type of meeting. It is not important to discuss here the different types of meetings exhaustively, but the reader will easily understand that the results emerging from a meeting will be different according to whether it is a decisional meeting for treatments, a team supervision about a difficult patient or a meeting to regulate team conflicts. Often interdisciplinary team meetings change into an indefinite patchwork with various objectives: for example, deciding on continuation of treatment, sharing about what has been difficult in the unit during the last few weeks, or informing about relational difficulties with patients' families.

8.6   Building a Common Vision and Sharing Leadership

In order to work as efficiently as possible within the interdisciplinary team, there is a need for building a common vision based on individual visions of the different team members. A common vision can be a fantastic motor for the team, as long as the team members as a group take time to think through the following questions: Which values do we share? What are our common objectives, meaning the objectives that we all can stick to together? As persons and as a group, which are our strong and weak points? How do we use our strong points complementarily for the patient's and his caregiver's benefit? How do we manage to remedy to our weak points?

According to Senge [9], a common vision is the answer to this question: What do we want to create together and how are we going to do so? It seems relatively evident that the preoccupations of the team are, or should be, centred on the patient's and caregiver's/family's quality of life. But it is less evident that the team also has to look at its own functioning. This requires that each team member is capable of reflective thinking and that the climate is stamped with authenticity, trust and humility, so that these issues can be shared.

Even if each profession can contribute equally to interdisciplinary teamwork, it is, however, not necessary that all members of the team are involved in all decisions. Cummings [10] notes that the decision-making process within the interdisciplinary team requires that the three following main questions should be asked:

1. Who has the information necessary to make decision? Before a decision can be made to send an immobile, oxygen-dependent patient home for a week-end, it is necessary to know if transport will be possible, if there are stairs that will be faced, how to arrange oxygen in the community, who will be able to stay with the patient and who will be available should things not work out. It is unlikely the chaplain or dietician, for example, would need to be involved in such a decision.

2. Who needs to be consulted before the decision is made? Using the above example, this decision requires consultation between the patient, his family, the physician, the nurse, and possibly the social worker and the community nurse. Failing to consult all those who will be implicated in carrying out the decision may mean that some important information is overlooked.

3. Who needs to be informed of a decision after it is made? In this example some of those needing to be informed might be the dietician (no meals on the unit for the week-end), administration (statistics, census) and community liaison (arranging ambulance transportation).

When aiming for the most adequate decisions to meet the needs and desires of patients and caregivers, according to the patients' health status, it is necessary to have efficient leadership within the team. Jackson [11] reminds us that the team leader has a vital role in this. As he is not the only person holding information, he knows who, within the team, is the best person to share information at one particular moment. The team leader does not have an answer to all questions, but he has to care about assuring his colleagues that the team is not alone in solving problems. Sharing leadership with participative management does not mean that everyone does everything at every moment. Hall and Weaver [12] mention that even if the responsibility is shared and collective, it is within the purview of the leader to identify the different developing steps and allow the team to take more and more

responsibility with progressive maturity. This means that the leader should have a wide knowledge of group dynamics, negotiation and conflict management, coping mechanisms, professional health and burnout prevention. His role will consist of recognising the personal and professional qualities of each member and encourage them to esteem each other, which will generate an atmosphere of enthusiasm and contagious motivation. As we mentioned at the beginning of this chapter, working as an interdisciplinary team has little precedent and it displaces the current, traditional hospital culture . This is why it is crucial that the different actors of the care scene learn to work together.

8.7 Learning Together to Work Together

The patient's bedside is a privileged place for learning interdisciplinarity, as is postgraduate education, especially if the group of participants in the course is composed of representatives of diverse professions. At the pre-graduate, continuing education and post-graduate levels, pluriprofessional training presents numerous advantages, highlighted in the WHO technical report 769 [13]:

- It teaches participants teamwork by promoting respect and mutual understanding between team members and allowing them to understand better each other's strong points, limits and functions.
- It contributes towards "decompartmentalising" the study programmes and prevents the creation of a caste system, which represents a barrier towards interprofessional collaboration.
- It allows the integration of diverse disciplines which have a role to play in health care, for example, health economy, sociology, communication science, computing, instruction and so on.
- It promotes pluriprofessional research, often in new or under-researched domains and guarantees an account of all pertinent aspects of any particular problem.

Education programs must insist on methods which allow team members to learn how to work efficiently together and to understand:
- The responsibility of the team as a group
- The role of each member in executing the team's mission
- The overlapping of the team members' roles
- The necessary processes for teamwork
- The role that the team plays in the global care system

It is precisely in the privileged space of the education setting that different professionals will be able to acquire such relational competencies. As Giordan [14] alludes, "to learn is to express oneself, because expression obliges each one to debate, to take in account the opposite opinions in order to elaborate another common explanation. Debating together the appropriate proposition to a problem leads to being able to back up one's position towards the initial conception, to strengthen one's reasoning and to reformulate one's ideas."

For this purpose, case study method represents an efficient pedagogical tool. As the care project gathers the team members, case study gathers learning professionals and obliges them to confront their ideas, because learning is defending one's point of view as long as it is pertinent and then letting it go when it is refuted. It is also about disputing opposing ideas and preparing a place for counterpropositions.

But in order that argumentation finds its place in the interdisciplinary dialogue, it seems essential that each profession is represented by one team member. Experience over the years has clearly shown this to be the case, especially in palliative care. According to Sebag-Lanoe [15], "palliative care training must necessarily include the interdisciplinary dimension, which represents one of the essential groundings for appropriate and coherent palliative care. This way, palliative medicine engenders re-invention of better co-ordinated institutional functioning, of wider inter-professional communication and of more efficient co-operation which can bring a significant benefice to the whole medical and nursing system. This reunification can and must begin through education."

In the future it will be essential that learning how to work in an interdisciplinary team not only represents a priority for the concerned actors, but also for the institutions where those actors work. In fact, there cannot be any pertinent learning if the enterprise, in this case the care institution, does not have a project of developing individual and collective professional competences. This means that the institution clearly takes a position for learning and developing interdisciplinary teamwork, not only in words but also in the concrete reality of daily practice. Poupart et al. [16] remind us that we do not practice interdisciplinarity in and of itself but because we judge that its contribution is necessary for improving the fate of individuals or society. Finally and primarily, the patient and his family should be the main beneficiary of the interdisciplinary teamwork, and the professionals should include them in a partner relationship as much as possible.

8.8   Conclusion

Interdisciplinary education and the validity of interdisciplinary work are part of a wider consideration concerning health costs and the constant search for efficiency in the quality of care offered to those with severe illness, as mentioned in the AACN Position Paper [17] regarding interdisciplinary education and practice. Among the competencies that are indispensable to practice interdisciplinarity, one may cite oral and written communication skills, problem-solving, understanding of human behaviours, development of values, all of which should enable the transition from a competitive to a collaborative mode. Let us note that collaborating means firstly having regard for one's own behaviour by asking oneself the following questions: Have I listened to the other person? Do I respect his values and his ideas which differ from mine? Do I know his field of action and do I recognise his competencies? Do I trust the other professional?

Not only does interdisciplinary collaboration bring undeniable benefit to the quality of services offered to patient and caregiver, but it is also a source of satisfaction for all professionals involved and thus represents a preventive element to professional burnout generated by difficult and complex situations. All health professionals—physician, nurse, pharmacist, social worker and others—agree that care co-ordination is vital for patient and caregivers. It is not as easy at it seems, and one must be clear that this interdisciplinary approach is meaningful only if it does not oppose each discipline's specificity, but on the contrary, joins it complementarily.

Living interdisciplinarity in daily practice is demanding. As Bolly et al. [18] describe, there is a need for each partner to keep the responsibility related to his own function and at the same time a need to recognise the different and complementary responsibilities of the other team members. Avoiding competitiveness, sharing information for the patient's benefit, co-ordinating and continually evaluating the team's functioning, and sharing ethical values are key elements for success. This is the price to pay so that interdisciplinary teamwork can topple the traditional organisation, at the level of individual actors as well as of health system, allowing each professional to take his place and fulfil his role. ---Let us hope that this interdisciplinary approach will, in the future, be part of all care settings, because each patient—no matter his pathology, the evolution of his disease or his life expectancy—deserves to benefit from global care, taking into account all dimensions of his and his family's/caregivers' suffering.

References

1.   1. Lassaunière JM, Plagès B (1995) Modèles organisationnels à l'hôpital, l'interdisciplinarité. Revue JALMALV 40:35–39
2.   2. Bolly C, Vanhalewyn M (2002) Aux sources de l'instant. Manuel de soins palliatifs à domicile. Weyrich, Neufchâteau, pp 193–201
3.   3. Saunders C (1994) Soins palliatifs, une approche pluridisciplinaire. Lamarre, Paris, p 7
4.   4. WHO (1990) Cancer pain relief and palliative care. Report of a World Health organization Expert Committee. Technical report series No. 804. World Health Organization, Geneva, p 21
5.   5. Le Boterf G (1998) L'ingénierie des compétences. Éditions d'Organisation, Paris, pp 68–69

6.   6. Société Française d'Accompagnement et de soins Palliatifs, Collège des acteurs en soins infirmiers (1999) L'infirmier(e) et les soins palliatifs. "Prendre soin": éthique et pratiques. Masson, Paris, p 11
7.   7. Girardier J (2001) Le travail en équipe de soins palliatifs. In: Jacquemin D (ed) Manuel de soins palliatifs. Dunod, Paris, p 371
8.   8. Drilling M (1997) L'interdisciplinarité comme processus d'apprentissage. J Croix-Rouge Suisse 3:12
9.   9. Senge P (1991) La cinquième discipline. First, Paris, p 264
10. 10. Cummings I (2003) The interdisciplinary team. In: Doyle D, Hanke G, MacDonald N (eds) Oxford textbook of palliative medicine, 2nd edn. Oxford University Press, New York, pp 19–30
11. 11. Jackson L (1994) Construire l'équipe. In Soins palliatifs, une approche pluridisciplinaire. Lamarre, Paris, pp 19–26
12. 12. Hall P, Weaver L (2001) Interdisciplinary education and teamwork: a long and winding road. Med Educ 35:872
13. 13. WHO (1988) Learning together to work together for health (World Health Organization Technical Report Series No. 769). World Health Organization, Geneva, p 17
14. 14. Giordan A (1998) Apprendre! Belin, Paris, pp 120–122
15. 15. Sebag-Lanoe R (1992) Les perspectives essentielles pour le développement de la formation en soins palliatifs. In: Roy DJ, Rapin CH (eds) Les défis (Amaryllis–les annales de soins palliatifs, vol 1). Clinical Research Institute of Montreal, Montréal, pp 77–82
16. 16. Poupart R, Simard J-J, Ouellet JP (1986) La création d'une culture organisationnelle, le cas des CLSC. FCLSQ , Montréal, p 32
17. 17. Larson E, DeBasio NO, Mundinger MO, Shoemaker JK (1995) AACN Position statement, interdisciplinary education and practice. http://www.aacn.nche.edu/Publications/positions/interdis.htm. Cited 19 September 2005
18. 18. Bolly C, Grandjean V, Vanhalewyn M, Vidal S (2003) L'éthique en chemin, démarche et créativité pour les soignants. Weyrich, Neufchâteau, pp 227–251

Bibliography

1. Annandale SJ, McCann S, Nattrass H, Regan de
    Bere S, Williams S, Evans D (2000) Achieving
    health improvements through interprofessional
    learning in south west England. J Interprof Care
    14:161–174
2. Forbes EJ, Fitzsimons V (1993) Education: the
    key to holistic interdisciplinary collaboration.
    Holist Nurs Pract 7:1–10
3. Gardebring S, Anderson L, Aroskar M, Benzie D,
    Zimmaro Bliss D, Cipolle R, Giebink GS, Hallin
    G, Keenan J, Weaver L (1996) Developing health
    care teams. A report by the Academic Health
    Center Task Force on Interdisciplinary Health
    Team Development. http://www.ahc.umn.edu/tf/
    ihtd.html. Cited 19 September 2005
4. Headrick LA, Wilcock PM, Batalden BP (1998)
    Interprofessional working and medical educa-
    tion. BMJ 316:771–774
5. Orchard CA, Curran V, Kabene S (2005) Creating
    a culture for interdisciplinary collaborative pro-
    fessional practice. Med Educ Online. http://www.
    med-ed-online.org/pdf/T0000063.pdf. Cited 9
    September 2005
6. Westberg J, Jason H (1993) Collaborative clinical
    education: the foundation of effective health care.
    Springer, Heidelberg Berlin New York

9 Cultural Aspects of Communication in Cancer Care

A. Surbone

Recent Results in Cancer Research, Vol. 168
© Springer-Verlag Berlin Heidelberg 2006

Summary

Cancer is increasing in incidence and prevalence worldwide, and the WHO has recently included cancer and its treatments as a health priority in developed and developing countries. The cultural diversity of oncology patients is bound to increase, and cultural sensitivity and competence are now required of all oncology professionals. A culturally competent cancer care leads to improved therapeutic outcome and it may decrease disparities in medical care. Cultural competence in medicine is a complex multilayered accomplishment, requiring knowledge, skills and attitudes whose acquisition is needed for effective cross-cultural negotiation in the clinical setting. Effective cultural competence is based on knowledge of the notion of culture; on awareness of possible biases and prejudices related to stereotyping, racism, classism, sexism; on nurturing appreciation for differences in health care values; and on fostering the attitudes of humility, empathy, curiosity, respect, sensitivity and awareness. Cultural competence in healthcare relates to individual professionals, but also to organizations and systems. A culturally competent healthcare system must consider in their separateness and yet in there reciprocal influences social, racial and cultural factors. By providing a framework of reference to interpret the external world and relate to it, culture affects patients' perceptions of disease, disability and suffering; degrees and expressions of concern about them; their responses to treatments and their relationship to individual physicians and to the healthcare system. Culture also influences the interpretation of ethical norms and principles, and especially of individual autonomy, which can be perceived either as synonymous with freedom or with isolation depending on the cultural context. This, in turn, determines the variability of truth-telling attitudes and practices worldwide as well as the different roles of family in the information and decision-making process of the cancer patient. Finally, culture affects individual views of the patient–doctor relationship in different contexts.

9.1 Introduction

The existence of major healthcare disparities in Western countries due to racial and socioeconomic factors and the presence of major differences in diverse groups with respect to key issues in healthcare have stirred intense debate and action in the medical, sociological and bioethical worlds. As a result, the notions of cultural sensitivity and of cultural competence have developed and have been increasingly applied to clinical medicine (Gostin1995; Kalnins 1997; Zweifler and Gonzalez 1998; Seibert et al. 2002). The acquisition of knowledge and skills in delivering culturally sensitive care became a requirement in medical schools in highly multiethnic societies such as the USA, where demographic projections estimate that minorities will grow from 29% in 2001 to almost 50% in 2050 (Seibert et al. 2002).

Delivering culturally sensitive cancer care is a priority for oncologists who are increasingly facing many ethical dilemmas arising from cross-cultural differences in their daily practices. Ethical issues in oncology are magnified by several factors: the severity of the illness and the negative metaphorical value of a cancer diagnosis; the physical and psychological suffering of the patient, at times extreme at the end of life; the impact of different degrees of social stigmatization and discrimination; the uncertainty related to the cancer prognosis and to the outcome and potential toxicity of experimental treatments; the side effects of many standard cancer therapies; and finally, the difficult balance between patients' desire to be involved in their care and their increased vulnerability due to the complex reality of cancer.

While the need for cultural competence may appear to be less acute in relatively more homogeneous societies and in countries with socialized healthcare systems, culture has profound implications in almost all contemporary societies because multiethnicity is increasingly common and because different cultures always co-exist within main cultures, as exemplified by the differences between North and South in many countries. Moreover, to the extent that both the patient and the physician always engage in an asymmetric yet reciprocal relationship, carrying their own personal and cultural identity, every clinical encounter and every patient–doctor relationship is an exercise in cultural competence (Surbone and Lowenstein 2003; Surbone 2004b).

Cultural differences between patients and healthcare professionals often give rise to some common bedside misunderstandings and conflicts with respect to truth telling, end-of-life choices, prevention and screening, and involvement in clinical trials. An example of the importance of cultural sensitivity in cancer care is the notion of "offering the truth" to cancer patients (Freeman 1993). This notion, based on allowing individual patients to choose their own paths and rhythm, was proposed as an effective means to respecting patients' autonomy to follow their own cultural norms.

In this chapter, I make frequent use of cross-cultural differences in truth telling as an illustration of the role of cultural competence in communication with cancer patients. In any patient–doctor relationship there is an inherent problem of what philosophers call act/object ambiguity, i.e. the fact that the truth of an assertion may refer either to the content or to the assertion

of the content. This is especially true when the appropriateness of an assertion needs to be evaluated in the context of particular circumstances, when a person may be right in what she says and may not be right in saying it in a given moment or in a given cultural context (Surbone 2002b). Giving blunt bad news to an uninformed cancer patient whose family has requested the physician not to do so is an example often encountered in multicultural oncology practices.

9.2 Culture and Medicine: Understanding Keywords

9.2.1 Culture

Culture is defined as the sum of the integrated patterns of knowledge, beliefs and behaviours of a given community (Olweny 1994). Cultural groups share thoughts, communication styles, ways of interacting, views of roles and relationships, values, practices, customs (Betancourt 2003). Culture is related to race and to ethnicity, and yet their domains are not superimposable. In essence, culture refers predominantly to the social, while race and ethnicity refer to the sociobiological domains (Betancourt et al. 2003; Kagawa-Singer 2003). We all belong simultaneously to multiple cultures, expressing themselves through specific languages, such as the medical one. Medicine is a culture that involves a specific language and is associated with a specific power position in most societies. As an example, both the patient and the doctor bring their culture(s) and language(s) to every clinical encounter (Surbone 2004b).

Factors such as socioeconomic status, educational level, spoken language, geographic areas, urban versus rural contexts, religion, gender, sexual orientation, occupation and disability define culture as well. All these nested elements of culture integrate as the woven threads of a tapestry to perform integrative and prescriptive functions, whose ultimate goal is to ensure the survival and well-being of its individual members (Kagawa-Singer 2003).

Culture contributes to our identity by providing a reference framework to interpret the external world and to relate to it, which has been described as a "web of significance" in which our daily lives are embedded (Swendson and Windsor 1996). This "web of significance" affects our perceptions of disease, disability and suffering; our degrees and expressions of concern about them; our responses to treatments; and our relationship to individual physicians and to the healthcare system (Seibert et al. 2002). Culture influences the meaning that each cancer patient gives to the suffering, and the loss of control and the many uncertainties that accompany their illness. The experience of cancer is a trial in the life of oncology patients, who often resort to the grand narratives provided by their own culture in order to interpret the physical and psychological pain of cancer (Nelson 1997). The different values that different persons attribute to suffering—whether of redemption, of punishment or of ill fate—are generally mediated by their culture. The patient and the physician must negotiate between their different views of illness and of health to achieve their common therapeutic goal (Kagawa-Singer and Blackhall 2001; Kagawa-Singer 2003)

The importance of cultural influences on our personal identity, however, should not be conceived in a deterministic way, as this only reinforces prejudicial and stereotyping attitudes that inevitably culminate in more or less overt forms of discrimination. In fact, there is constant redefinition of cultural identity. Cultures are dynamic, interdependent and fluid, and they evolve from within as well as under the reciprocal influence of other cultures. Members of different racial, ethnic and cultural groups undergo assimilation and acculturation. Individual persons or groups do not always conform to their own culture, and cultural identity is only a dimension of one's personal identity. When we make generalizations that are not fully substantiated by evidence, we fail to recognize that cultural identity is not a substitute for personal identity, which is rather primarily grounded in one's own experiences in life as well as in universal human values (Surbone 2004b).

Furthermore, the progressive exposure to global communication and the increasing demographic mobility determine rapid cultural changes in contemporary societies, to the point that cultural identity today goes well beyond geographic and ethnic boundaries. The risk of such globalization is that the Western model, however, would prevail over deeply routed cultural beliefs in a sort of cultural hegemony (Surbone 2003a , 2004b). On the contrary, different cultural identities are a welcome reality of our world, where some cultures continue to privilege individual autonomy, while others are more family- and community-centred. Thus, both cultural differences and cultural similarities need to be acknowledged and respected also in medicine, where personal and cultural sensitivity and competence are equally needed. In oncology practice, as an example, we can now find striking cross-cultural similarities in the approach of cancer patients to the salient moments in the course of their illness, such as when facing end-of-life decisions (Kagawa-Singer and Blackhall 2001).

9.2.2 Cultural Sensitivity

Cultural sensitivity for healthcare workers has been defined as their being "sensitive to the ways in which community members' values and perceptions about healthcare differ from their own" (Zweifler and Gonzalez 1998). Cultural sensitivity is based on the recognition of cultural diversity and on the avoidance of stereotyping, but also common universal similarities beyond cultural differences. It describes attitudes, values, beliefs and personal insight of healthcare professionals, including openness to and curiosity about cultural differences. By contrast, cultural awareness relates to the healthcare professional's knowledge of those areas of cultural expression which mostly affect patients' views on healthcare matters such as language, kinship patterns, religion, and special dietary habits (Doorenbos et al. 2005).

9.2.3 Cultural Competence

Cultural competence in healthcare not only relates to individual professionals but also to organizations and systems.(Kalnins 1997; Betancourt et al. 2003). A culturally competent healthcare system "acknowledges and incorporates—at all levels—the importance of culture, assessment of cross-cultural relations, vigilance toward the dynamics that result form cultural differences, expansion of cultural knowledge, and adaptation of services to meet culturally unique needs" of patients or groups of patients (Betancourt et al. 2003). A culturally competent healthcare system must also consider in their separateness and yet in their reciprocal influences social, racial and cultural factors. In understanding and trying to overcome the causes for major healthcare disparities in many Western countries, it has become evident that cultural variations in patients' health beliefs, values, preferences, and behaviours affect the recognition of symptoms, the threshold for seeking care, and the willingness and ability to communicate and explain symptoms, as well as the understanding of standard information about diagnosis, prognosis and treatment options, the trust in different professionals and the adherence to prescribed treatments (Betancourt 2003). Clearly, these are all essential elements of oncology care—a practice that can no longer exist without cultural competence.

9.3   Teaching Cultural Competence to Clinicians

Cultural competence in medicine is thus a complex multilayered accomplishment. It requires knowledge, skills and attitudes whose acquisition is needed for effective cross-cultural negotiation in the clinical setting. A culturally competent cancer care will lead to improved therapeutic outcome and it may decrease disparities in medical care (Langer 1999; Stewart et al. 1999; Betancourt et al. 2003, Vega 2005). The difficulty of establishing exactly what cultural competence entails for the clinician and the failure of many programmes to really teach about one's culture as well as about other cultures has recently been highlighted. Involving medical students and physician in training in early programmes that will help them understand first their own cultural framework is most important (Fox 2005). This includes understanding the Western culture of medicine and exploring possible biases and prejudices (Newmann 1988).

There are different methods for teaching cultural competence. The "multicultural approach" focuses on providing relevant information about different cultures with respect to different health issues. In oncology, as an example, cultural competence entails a basic knowledge of different cultural practices of truth telling throughout the world, as I illustrate in the next section. Another method, the "cross-culturally based systems approach", focuses on the individual patient as a teacher and on the multiple variables involved in the process of communication. It presupposes the physician's awareness of his/her own cultural beliefs and values, and it aims at the development of attitudes and clinical skills (Betancourt et al. 2003).

Effective cultural competence is based on increasing physicians' knowledge of the concept of culture as well as of the key notions related to culture, such as stereotyping, racism, classism, sexism; on nurturing appreciation for differences in healthcare values; and finally on fostering the attitudes of humility, empathy, curiosity, respect, sensitivity and awareness (Kagawa-Singer 2003). These attitudes, however, are in no way confined to cross-cultural clinical encounters but rather are essential to all physicians and healthcare professionals.

Some unsolved issues related to the teaching and acquisition of cultural competence have recently been analysed in the medical literature. First, most cultural competence programmes are limited to a brief training. Second, comprehensive strategies including individual and also organizational changes require both commitment and resources that are still scarce. Third, there is lack of formal consensus on a clear definition of cultural competence and what the contents of its teaching should be. Finally, research-based empirical evidence on the effectiveness of cultural competence is still missing (Vega 2005).

Despite the difficulties inherent in teaching the complexity of cultural competence, the field has made major progress since it was born approximately 20 years ago. In the USA accreditations bodies such as the Commission on Accreditation of Hospital Organizations require mandatory training in cultural competence for licensure of healthcare professionals (Betancourt 2003; Vega 2005).

9.4 Evolution and Persistence of Cross-cultural Differences in Truth Telling: A Paradigmatic Illustration

Truth telling is central to communication between the patient and the doctor in clinical medicine and especially in oncology. Truth telling is also a core issue in bioethics, as it relates to the doctrines of informed consent and of cultural competence. The debate on truth telling has always been particularly intense in oncology and it has greatly influenced other domains of medicine.

The doctrine of informed consent was born in 1947 as a result of the Nuremberg Trial. One of the first milestone studies of truth telling practices in the USA showed that 10% of surveyed physicians would never reveal a cancer diagnosis (Oken 1961). By contrast, over the following two decades, physicians' truth-telling practices in the USA changed dramatically and in the late 1970s 98% of surveyed US physicians revealed the cancer diagnosis to their patients (Novack 1979). Truth telling and informed consent were a reflection of the growing Anglo-American emphasis on individual autonomy, grounded in a strong tradition of privacy rights and personal liberty (Beauchamp and Childress 1994).

In other cultural contexts and within multiethnic minorities in the USA, truth telling attitudes and practices were rarely discussed until the late 1980s and early 1990s (Holland et al. 1987; Surbone 1992; Mystadikou et al. 1996). The initial debate on truth telling was followed by a wealth of reports from different countries, suggesting major cross-cultural differences in truth telling (Surbone and Zwitter 1997). In countries centred on family and community values, the word "autonomy" was often perceived more as synonymous with "isolation" than with "freedom". Those societies have a more paternalistic vision of the patient–doctor relationship and they attribute a protective role to families and physicians with respect to the ill person (Surbone 1992; Mystadikou et al. 2004). Painful medical truths were often withheld or strongly mitigated to avoid taking away hope from the cancer patient or causing her severe distress. In most cases, physicians only informed the patients' families, while keeping the patient in the dark. Often this resulted in a "conspiracy of silence" where doctors and relatives were often caught in the web of half-truths that in many cases left the patient suffering alone, unable to ask questions and find answers, often even deprived of the chance to put in order their affairs or to say good-bye to their loved ones (Surbone 1992).

A recent worldwide shift in the understanding of the patient–doctor relationship has resulted in a rapid evolution of truth-telling attitudes among patients and physicians. The practice of truth telling to cancer patients is now increasingly common and public polls conducted through the media in different countries show a parallel shift in public opinion in favour of more open disclosure of the truth to cancer patients (Harrison et al. 1997; Seo et al. 2000; Mystadikou et al. 2004; Surbone et al. 2004).

Different medical, legal and societal factors, all intertwined, have contributed to the evolution of truth-telling attitudes and practices in oncology throughout the world. These main factors appear to be very similar to those that influenced the shift from non-disclosure to disclosure in the USA between the 1960s and the 1980s (Novack 1979; Anderlick et al. 2000. Patients of different cultural backgrounds have started demanding respect of their rights, including that of sharing any decision making about their health and illnesses, and physicians have changed their practices of disclosure. As a result of the contributions of physicians, patients, the public and the media, the word "cancer" seems to have lost some of its metaphorical implications related to imminent and inevitable death, and cancer patients suffer less stigmatization and isolation.

Despite the international trend just described, partial disclosure and non-disclosure are still supported and practiced by physicians throughout the world. Studies suggest that even among those physician who assert that patients have a right to be informed, the actual rate of disclosure remains low (Grassi et al. 2000; Tse et al. 2003, Monge and Sotomayor 2004; Surbone et al. 2004; Voogt et al. 2005). Also, surveys of cancer patients reveal a persistent lack of awareness of the severity and curability of their illness

(IGEO 1999). These data may be interpreted as a function of anthropological and sociocultural differences. For example, cultural changes may occur in cohorts related to social and attitudinal changes of different generations (Glenn 1980). Also, partial disclosure may still occur in those cultural contexts where the requirement for a substantive consent allows doctors to separate the medical act from the reasons behind it, or where abiding to traditional family and community values may take priority over following the written law (Surbone et al. 2004). Paternalism may be an expression of traditional hierarchical and authoritarian values that still predominate in specific geographic areas historically less exposed to the Western model.

Variations in patients' and physicians' attitudes and practices, however, may also be related to age, geographic location and the type of treating institution in almost all countries. There are similar observed differences in disclosure and information rates in urban versus rural communities and in northern versus southern areas of different countries. Also, major variations have been reported among patients and physicians in leading teaching institutions and large city hospitals versus private and peripheral practices, regardless of the country (Baile et al. 2002).

According to extensive data from the Anglo-American world, including Australia, Canada, the UK and the USA, most patients expect truthfulness about their illness and wish to participate to the decision-making process involving their treatments (Emanuel et al. 2004) In Western countries, more informed and more involved patients seem to fare better in terms of compliance with difficult therapies, and sharing the decision-making process between the patient and the doctor seems to result in better care and better outcomes (Baile et al. 2002; Fallowfield and Jenkins 2004 ; Katz et al. 2005; Nattinger 2005; Brown et al. 2004).

Recent data collected from the growing number of patients who are now informed of their cancer diagnosis in countries where traditionally the truth was withheld seem to confirm that these patients also do not experience particular distress or discomfort when they are told the truth about their cancer (Elwyn et al. 2002). Furthermore, studies on patient preferences seem to suggest strong similarities with Western types in terms of patients' general needs and preferences for communication (Sekimoto et al. 2004 ; Nayak et al. 2005).

9.5   Culturally Competent Care and Respect for Autonomy

The increased emphasis on personal self-governance in the Anglo-American world is mirrored in the current model of the patient–doctor relationship, which includes doctors' moral obligation to respect and foster their patients' autonomy and to develop equal partnerships with them, first and foremost through the practice of truth telling. The autonomy model is in sharp contradistinction to the paternalistic model of charismatic physicians who, at their discretion, maintain all power, including that of withholding truth (Beauchamp and Childress 1994).

However, the current Western preoccupation with equality and autonomy, uniformity and impartiality, with rules and reciprocity suited for the voluntarily bargaining relations of non-intimate equals often fails to capture the essence of the patient–doctor relationship (Surbone and Lowenstein 2003). This is an asymmetrical relation of help between the patient, who is in a "uniquely dependent state" by virtue of her illness, and the physician who assumes the responsibility to care for the patient (Pellegrino and Thomasma 1988). The patient–doctor relationship thus carries particular ethical implications related to vulnerability, asymmetry, distance and intimacy, which require considerations of care, trust and justice along with respect for relational autonomy (Baier 1994; Sherwin 1998; Anderlick 2000).

The notion of "respect for the patient's relational autonomy" is very helpful in framing the issue of truth telling and in trying to analyse different attitudes and practices. It is also necessary to understand the many unsolved aspects of truth telling that go beyond cultural differences. "Autonomy" is a complex concept, as it refers to the one's capacity to choose, but also to the ability to implement one's choices. Autonomy is a necessary attribute of rational human beings and it is universally valid (Mahowald 2000). However, both internal and external factors and resources contribute to one's autonomy and from the beginning to the end of our lives, we are embedded in a context of social relations, which shape us and sustain us (Sherwin 1998). Regardless of one's cultural identity, autonomy is always relational and situated, rather than simply a matter of individual choice. Imposing the truth onto an unprepared patient whose cultural expectation is to be shielded from painful medical truths is not necessarily an act of respect for autonomy (Pellegrino 1992). Any patient should be free to delegate her autonomy to a certain extent to the physician or the family and the community, when this corresponds to her individual or cultural value system.

Finally, in clinical medicine one cannot ignore the actual sociocultural conditions that make the patient's autonomy possible. As an example, the patient's decision to participate in a clinical trial often does not depend only on the information about the trial, but it is also influenced by socioeconomic barriers to access (Brawley 2003). In the field of genetic screening, the decision to seek genetic information is in large part a function of social perceptions and discriminatory practices, which may greatly limit one's autonomy .

9.6 Common Cross-cultural Issues in Bedside Oncology

9.6.1 Communication About Diagnosis

There is ample evidence that the diagnosis of cancer is now being revealed to most patients in many, if not most, countries. In a survey of 167 oncologists attending the 1999 International Meeting of the American Society of Clinical Oncology, there was no difference between Western and non-Western physicians in disclosure of diagnosis (Baile et al. 2002). By contrast, whether and how to disclose prognosis and to deliver "bad news" is far from being a settled issue even in those countries with a long tradition of truth telling (Butow et al. 1996; Parker et al. 2001; Baile et al. 2002).

The cancer diagnosis, even when complex and difficult, can be established and confirmed with good degrees of certainty that can be conveyed to the patient, though specific modalities of com-

munication may be culturally determined. In many cultures, for instance, doctors often use euphemisms, such as "growth" or "condition" instead of the word "cancer" and patients prefer them, even when they wish to be told the truth (Baile et al. 2002). In some cultures, the utterance of words bearing a negative connotation is believed to affect the reality for worse (Carrese and Rhodes 1995). In other cultures, words such as "cancer" or "depression" do not exist, and people do not share our Western causal explanations. In a poignant essay, Dr. Levy from Zimbabwe reported that her patients perceived cancer as a ghost (Levy 1997). In all cultures, but particularly in those where patients are shielded from open truth telling, non-verbal communication is extremely important (Dunn et al. 1993). As the meaning of non-verbal forms of communication is subject to great cultural variability, oncology professionals practicing in multicultural settings need to have some specific knowledge of cross-cultural differences in non-verbal communication. Pauses and silences always have tremendous effect on our patients, and we know that almost any piece of information can be downplayed or emphasized through body gestures, eye contact and modulation of one's tone of voice. The effect of pauses and gestures, however, is not the same universally. As an example, in most Anglo- and Latin-American cultures, some form of touch from one's physician is generally equated with an expression of empathy. The degree of physical closeness that patients expect and desire, on the contrary, appears to be very different in Asian cultures (Ammann and Baumgarten 2005; Fujimori et al. 2005).

9.6.2 Communication About Prognosis and Risk Assessment

When talking with their patients about prognosis and risk assessment, physicians are acutely confronted with the interplay of certainty and uncertainty at the cognitive level, and of hope and expectations at the psychological and spiritual level (Del Vecchio et al. 1990; Surbone 1997; Clayton et al. 2005 ; Chochinov et al. 2005; Ferrell 2005; Hagerty et al. 2005; Hartmann 2005; Kalemkerian 2005). Many recent studies confirm that the balance between fostering and taking away hope is a very delicate one, and that many physicians may be reluctant to be involved in any discourse on hope. These issues are extensively discussed in other chapters in this book, by Drs. Stiefel and Razavi and by Dr. Lloyd, who addresses specifically communication in palliative care and at the end of life.

Many of the difficulties encountered by patients and physicians alike in discussing prognosis seem to go beyond cultural differences. Even in Anglo-American cultures, the disclosure of prognostic information occurs much less often and it is left to the individual physician, while the disclosure of diagnosis is required by law (Spiro 2005). Often, patients specifically ask not to be kept informed of the details of their diseases, but sometimes it is the physician who does not feel comfortable taking away too much hope from patients.

Prognostication is related to the physician's awareness of the asymmetry and power imbalance inherent in the patient–doctor relationship—something that is universally true, and yet may deserve greater consideration in different cultural contexts. Bye the patient–doctor relationship is an asymmetric relationship, where the vulnerability that the illness creates in the patient meets the expertise of the physician whose help has been requested by the patient. In a relation of help, the power is not equally distributed between the partners, and abuses may occur in different forms. To avoid such more or less subtle abuses of power within the patient–doctor relationship, it is essential for the physician to acknowledge its intrinsic asymmetry as well as the uncertainties of clinical medicine (Surbone and Lowenstein 2003; Howe 2003). As an example, physicians at times may hide behind statistic information to maintain control in the patient–doctor relationship or to mask their own difficulties in accepting their own limitations with respect to the possibility of cure. A profound sense of humility and respect for the patient as "Other", accompanied by individual and cultural sensitivity, may facilitate effective communication about prognosis and about risk assessment (Surbone 2005).

9.6.3 Role of Families

Cancer is an illness that not only affects the sick person, but also their entire family, and the healing and caring process depend also on the interactions of the physician with the family and the community (Baider et al. 2000). The internal dynamics of the family are inevitably altered by the cancer illness and by the caregiving responsibilities that families take upon themselves, especially at the end of life. In almost all cultures, women tend to be the caregivers in the family (Surbone 2003b; Mook et al. 2003; Baider et al. 2000). The relationship with the patient's family is amply discussed by Dr. Firth in this book, and I will thus only briefly treat some cultural aspects.

Families are almost always involved in the course of the evolution of the patient's cancer in every culture, and they are rarely be excluded from participating in the process of information and communication, unless it is the expressed wish of the patient (Farber et al. 1999). The extent and modalities of family involvement are different and in some countries families make decisions in place of uninformed patients. In many countries, especially in Asia, the family is always consulted before revealing a cancer diagnosis to the patient (Seo et al. 2000; Kagawa-Singer and Blackhall 2001). Although most patients in the USA believe that the patient should be the primary decision maker, still major differences were reported in African-Americans and white patients and their families (Phipps et al. 2003).

Often, it is the family that requests the hospital staff not to disclose the truth to the patient, also in countries with strict requirements for informed consent (Kinsella 2001; Anderlick et al. 2000 ; Baile et al. 2002; Elwyn et al. 2002; Phipps et al. 2003). In a recent study of a multicultural patient population attending a large cancer centre, particular emphasis was placed on tailoring the degree of information given to different patients in view of their individual but also family and community values, especially when dealing with specific requests to withhold or to mitigate the truth (Anderlick et al. 2000). In Western countries, it has been reported that the intervention of relatives almost invariably renders much more complicated the discussions between the patient and the physician (Higginson and Costantini 2002).

A 2005 survey of 150 relatives of recently diagnosed cancer patients in Turkey revealed that 66% did not want the diagnosis to be revealed to the patient. Factors that influenced the family request not to tell were male gender of the patient, diagnosis other than breast cancer, stage IV disease, insufficient family knowledge about cancer in general, strong religious beliefs and the absence of the patient's request for disclosure (Ozdogan et al. 2004). Negotiating the concerns of family members while respecting patients' needs in terms of information and shared decision making can be extremely challenging (Benson and Britten 1996).There may in fact be distinct informational needs to be addressed (Clayton et al. 2005). Families may require guidance and support when faced with a tell or not tell situation (Maguire and Faulkner 1988; Maguire et al. 1996). Furthermore, patients, family caregivers and physicians all interact in a connected system and efforts are needed to improve understanding and concordance among them (Farber et al. 2003).

9.6.4 Respecting Cultural Differences in Western Hospital Settings

Respect for cultural differences and for relational autonomy does not have to be blind, nor does it require that physicians subscribe to any form of cultural determinism. Physicians, while being sensitive to and avoiding any form of stereotyping and/or of cultural imperialism, are entitled to advocate for their patients' rights to self-determination. Often, the lack of information conveyed arises from miscommunication or real conflicts between the patient and the family and the physicians' role is to clarify such misunderstanding by being on the patient's side (Clayton et al. 2005). In the clinical setting, physicians foster their patients' autonomy by always putting their patient first and by spending the necessary time to understand what their patients wishes are in truth-telling matters.

Respecting different attitudes toward truth telling of patients treated in a society with a homogenous medico-legal system, in which withholding the truth is considered an infringement on the patient's autonomy, poses major quandaries

(Anderlick et al. 2000; Surbone 2003). In the contemporary Western healthcare context, uninformed patients tend be a source of stress for the hospital staff, and lack of information can be an obstacle to good medical care (Fallowfield and Jenkins 1999). It is not advisable to encourage physicians to go against the deontologic and legal requirements of their society. While it may be possible—though no longer recommendable—to withhold some information from cancer patients in countries where this is a commonly accepted practice based on ethically justified norms, it is always a mistake not to be truthful to cancer patients treated in a country where disclosure is the ethical norm and it is legally required. In the course of a chronic illness such as cancer, entailing frequent visits to different specialists and often requiring periods of hospitalization, almost all patients will inevitably be told the truth at some point and consequently lose trust in the treating physicians and team (Fallowfield et al. 2002). Often, in fact, disclosure occurs through staff members, who may not have an established connection with the patients and may be unaware that relevant information had been withheld.

Cross-cultural medical encounters pose many additional difficulties related to language and therefore to the process of translation. Studies in philosophy and anthropology have established that language goes far beyond semantics, and rather it reflects different peoples' ways of life. These, in turn, are based on different meanings and values that are acquired within one's culture. In acquiring language skills, people from early ages learn about the truth-value of different assertions in a specific cultural context (Williams 2002). Translations from a language into another are thus very complex and require particular care when they involve the delivery of medical information and of bad news (Russell Searight and Gafford 2005).

9.6.5 Improving Effective Communication in Cross-cultural Medical Encounters

Establishing rigid guidelines for cross-cultural encounters is a difficult task. Excellent studies have suggested steps that may be followed in cross-cultural patient–doctor encounters (Kagawa-Singer 2003). Following are recommendations based on my own clinical experience and research in cross-cultural encounters with cancer patients (Surbone 2004a). Healthcare professionals should not make assumptions based on race, nationality or language of their patients, and rather they should take the time to ask them to briefly describe their cultural background, including their religious beliefs. Though it may appear superfluous, it is often appropriate for physicians of a different culture to briefly acknowledge their own background.

Physicians should also ask new patients to what type of family they belong—whether extended or nuclear, close or distant—and ask them directly to what extent they wish their family or friends to be involved. In any cross-cultural encounter, the physician should tactfully and yet openly ask patients how informed they wish to be about their illness and to investigate their information preference, while also clarifying that he or she must respect the laws of the country of practice (Butow et al. 1997).

With respect to translation, it often helps to inquire with the patient about the language spoken at home. Professional translation, when available, should always be offered and the translator should be considered and involved also as a "cultural mediator". When the translation is performed by a relative or a friend, the physician should find a way to double-check at random if the translation is correct or if it leaves out relevant information (Russell Searight and Gafford 2005).

Finally, during the course of a chronic illness that often progresses through many phases, it is essential to verify the patient's understanding of the illness at different points. This can be done by occasionally pausing to let the patients verbalize their grasp of the situation as well as their concerns and hopes. Listening and observing become equally important in cross-cultural encounters where language barriers are frequent.

9.7 Conclusions

This chapter has treated the most relevant cultural aspects of communication in cancer care.

Cultural competence is about the cultural differences and also the cross-cultural similarities that exist within the context of good communication in the clinic. Communication is an art that requires dispositions and virtues, as well as experience and training. Multiple studies have confirmed that communication skills can be taught and learned by physicians at any stage of their career. Being a good and effective communicator helps both physicians and their patients and families. Learning how to break bad news, how to deal with an angry or difficult patient, how to approach end-of-life discussions with cancer patients is essential to oncology professionals, including the most empathic and compassionate ones, who need a solid framework within which to best communicate with their patients as well as to prevent burn-out in their personal lives.

As an experiential skill, communication can and should be taught with different methodologies that have been shown to improve physicians' communication skills as well as patients' satisfaction. These subjects are extensively treated by Drs. Fallowfield and Jenkins and by Drs. Favre, Despland and Stiefel in this book. Being a good communicator, however, also involves the moral character of the physician and requires individual and cultural sensitivity, empathy and compassion, respect for the "other" in front of us and genuine interest in what she has to say and in how she feels (Spiro 1993; Butow et al. 1996; Fox 2005; Surbone 2005). A good communicator never betrays the complexity of the patient–doctor relationship and of the cultural differences and similarities that deeply affect any communication process.

In my own experience of over 20 years of practicing medical oncology in different countries and multicultural settings, I have become convinced that rarely are our patients unaware of their own situation, because they are the ones who suffer from the illness and from the cancer treatments with their immediate and long-term sequelae. Communication of the truth is always possible during the course of a long-lasting patient–doctor relationship. Yet, clinical algorithms and guidelines for optimal communication are difficult to establish and they are not necessarily applicable cross-culturally. Furthermore, acquiring and practicing cultural competence can often fail to produce a measurable impact on the delivery of healthcare, especially when it represents the isolated effort of individual healthcare professionals and does not reach and overcome organizational and structural barriers (Betancourt et al. 2003).

Culturally competent cancer care requires knowledge, dedication and time. Oncology professionals are increasingly working under financial and time constraints and often under enormous peer pressure. Yet, delivering culturally competent cancer care has not only become a necessity, but is also an extremely rewarding task. Nurturing the profound sense of privilege, enrichment and fulfilment that derives from meeting uniquely different patients is essential to our ability to care for our patients and also for our inner life as physicians and oncology professionals. Those of us who have been gifted with occasional epiphanies of real communication with our patients know only too well the importance of sharing a unique moment of intimacy or of deep connection with them, even beyond what we consider good standard communication (Matthews et al. 1993; Lowenstein 1997). While these epiphanies may be increasingly rare in today's Western healthcare systems, where patient care is often fragmented and rushed, cultural sensitivity and cultural competency contribute to the ability of oncology professionals to reach deeper levels of communication with their patients and to help them cope effectively with the many challenges of cancer.

References

1. Ammam RA, Baumgarten L (2005) Bad news in oncology: which are the right words? Supp Care Cancer 13:275–276
2. Anderlik MR, Pentz RD, Hess KR. Revisiting the truth telling debate: a study of disclosure practices at a major cancer center. J Clin Ethics 11:251–259
3. Back AL, Arnold RM, Baile WF et al. (2005) Approaching different communication tasks in oncology. CA Cancer J Clin 55:164–177
4. Baider L, Cooper CL, De-Nour K (2000) Cancer and the family, 2nd edn. J. Wiley & Sons, Sussex
5. Baier A (1994) Moral prejudices. Essays on ethics. Harvard University Press, Cambridge
6. Baile WF, Lenzi R, Parker PA et al. (2002) Oncologists' attitudes toward and practices in giving bad news: an exploratory study. J Clin Oncol 20:2189–2196
7. Beauchamp T, Childress JF (1994) Principles of biomedical ethics, 4th edn. Oxford University Press, New York
8. Benson J, Britten N (1996) Respecting the autonomy of cancer patients when talking with their families: qualitative analysis of semistructured interviews with patients. BMJ 313:729–731
9. Betancourt JR (2003) Cross-cultural medical education: conceptual approaches and frameworks for evaluation. Acad Med 78:560–569
10. Betancourt JR, Green AR, Carrillo JE, Ananeh-Firempong II O (2003) Defining cultural competence: a practical framework for addressing racial/ethnic disparities in health and health care. Public Health Rep 188:293–302
11. Blackhall L (1995) Ethnicity and attitudes toward patient autonomy. JAMA 274:820–825
12. Brawley OW (2003) Population categorization and cancer statistics. Cancer Metastasis Rev 22:11–19
13. Brown RF, Butow PN, Sharrock MA et al. (2004) Education and role modelling for clinical decisions with female cancer patients. Health Expect 7:303–316
14. Butler L, Degner L, Baile W et al. (2005) Developing communication competency in the context of cancer: a critical interpretive analysis of provider training programs. Psycho-oncology 14:861–872
15. Butow PN, Kazemi JN, Beeney LJ et al. (1996) When the diagnosis is cancer: patient communication experiences and preferences. Cancer 77:2630–2637
16. Butow PN, Maclean M, Dunn SM (1997) The dynamics of change: cancer patients' preferences for information, involvement and support. Ann Oncol 8:857–863
17. Carrese J, Rhodes L (1995) Western bioethics on the Navajo reservation: benefit or harm? JAMA 274:826–829
18. Cherny NL, Coyle N, Foley KM (1994) Suffering in the advanced cancer patient: a definition and taxonomy. J Palliat Care 10:57–70
19. Chochinov HM, Hack T, Hassard T et al. (2005) Dignity therapy: a novel psychotherapeutic intervention for patients near the end of life. J Clin Oncol 23:5520–5525

20. Clayton JM, Butow PN, Tattersall MHN (2005) The needs of terminally ill patients versus those of caregivers for information regarding prognosis and end of life issues. Cancer 103:1957–1964

21. Del Vecchio Good MJ, Good BJ et al. (1990) American oncology and the discourse on hope. Cult Med Psychiatry 14:59–79

22. Doorenbos AZ, Meyers Schim S, Benkert R, Borse NN (2005) Psychometric Evaluation of the cultural competence assessment instrument among healthcare providers. Nurs Res 54 :324–331

23. Dunn SM, Patterson PU, Butow PN et al. (1993) Cancer by another name: a randomized trial of the effects of euphemism and uncertainty in communicating with cancer patients. J Clin Oncol 11:989–996

24. Elwyn TS, Fetters MD, Sasaki H, Tsuda T (2002) Responsibility and cancer disclosure in Japan. Soc Sci Med 54:281–293

25. Emanuel EJ, Fairclough DL, Eolfe P, Emanuel LL (2004) Talking with terminally ill patients and their caregivers about death, dying and bereavement. Is it stressful? Is it helpful? Arch Intern Med 164:1999–2004

26. Fallowfield L, Jenkins V (1999) Effective communication skills are the key to good cancer care. Eur J Cancer 35:1592–1597

27. Fallowfield L, Jenkins V (2004) Communicating sad, bad, difficult news in medicine. Lancet 363:312–319

28. Fallowfield LJ, Jenkins VA, Beveridge HA (2002) Truth can hurt but deceit hurts more: communication in palliative care. Palliat Med 16:297–303

29. Farber SJ, Egnew TR, Herman-Bertsch JL (1999) Issues in end-of-life care: family practice faculty perceptions. J Fam Pract 49:525–530

30. Farber SJ, Egnew TR, Herman-Bertsch JL et al. (2003) Issues in end-of-life care: patient, caregiver and clinical perceptions. J Palliat Med 6:19–31

31. Ferrell B (2005) Dignity therapy: advancing the science of spiritual care in terminal illnesses. J Clin Oncol 23:5427–5428

32. Fox RC (2005) Cultural competence and the culture of medicine. New Engl J Med 353:1316–1319

33. Freeman B (1993) Offering truth. One ethical approach to the uninformed cancer patient. Arch Intern Med 153:572–576

34. Fujimori M, Akechi T, Azikuki N et al. (2005) Good communication with patients receiving bad news about cancer in Japan. Psycho-oncology 14:1043–1051

35. Gostin LO (1995) Informed consent, cultural sensitivity and respect for persons. JAMA 274:844–845

36. Glenn ND (1980) Values, attitudes and beliefs. In: Brim OG, Kagan (eds) Constancy and change in human development. Harvard University Press, Cambridge MA, pp 596–640

37. Grassi L, Giraldi T, Messina EG et al. (2000) Physicians' attitudes to and problems with truth-telling to cancer patients. Supp Care Cancer 8:40–45

38. Hagerty RG, Butow PN, Ellis PM et al. (2005) Communicating with realism and hope: incurable cancer patients' views on disclosure of prognosis. J Clin Oncol 23:1278–1288

39. Harrison A, Al-Saadi AMH, Al-Kaabi ASO et al. (1997) Should doctors inform terminally ill patients? The opinions of nationals and doctors in the United Arab Emirates. J Med Ethics 23:101–107

40. Hartmann LC (2005) Unrealistic expectations. J Clin Oncol 23:4231–4232

41. Higginson IJ, Costantini M (2002) Communication in the end of life care: a comparison of team assessment in three European countries. J Clin Oncol 20:3674–3682

42. Holland JC, Geary N, Marchini A, Tross S (1987) An international survey of physician attitudes and practices in regard to revealing the diagnosis of cancer. Cancer Invest 5:151–154

43. Howe EG (2003) Overcoming the downside of asymmetry. J Clinic Ethics 14:137–151

44. Hudelson P, Stalder H (2005) Sociocultural diversity and medical education. Rev Med Suisse 1:2214–2217

45. IGEO—The Italian Group for the Evaluation of Outcomes in Oncology (1999) Awareness of disease among Italian cancer patients: Is there a need for further improvement in patient information? Ann Oncol 10:1095–1100

46. Kagawa-Singer M (2003) A strategy to reduce cross-cultural miscommunication and increase the likelihood of improving health outcomes. Acad Med 78:577–587

47. Kagawa-Singer M, Blackhall LJ (2001) Negotiating cross-cultural issues at the end of life. JAMA 286:2993–3001

48. Kalemkerian GP (2005) Commentary on "unrealistic expectations". J Clin Oncol 23:4233–4234

49. Kalnins ZP (1997) Cultural diversity and today's managed health care. J Cult Diversity 4:43

50. Katz SJ, Lantz PM, Janz NK et al. (2005) Patient involvement in surgery treatment decisions for breast cancer. J Clin Oncol 23 :5526–5533

51. Kinsella L (2001) Truth telling in patient care. Resolving ethical issues. Nursing 12:52–55

52. Langer N (1999) Culturally competent professionals in therapeutic alliances enhance patient compliance. J Health Care Poor Underserved 10:19–26

53. Levy LM (1997) Communication with the cancer patient in Zimbabwe. Ann NY Acad Sci 809:133–141

54. Lowenstein J (1997) The midnight meal and other essays about doctors, patients and medicine. Yale University Press, New Haven London

55. Maguire P, Faulkner A (1988) Communicate with cancer patients: handing uncertainty, collusion, denial. BMJ 297:972–974

56. Maguire P, Faulkner A, Booth K et al. (1996) Helping cancer patients disclose their concerns. Eur J Cancer 32:78–81

57. Mahowald MB (2000) Genes, women, equality. Oxford University Press, New York Oxford

58. Maltoni M, Caraceni A, Brunelli C et al. (2005) Prognostic factors in advanced cancer patients: evidence-based clinical recommendations. A study by the Steering Committee of the European Association for Palliative Care. J Clin Oncol 23:6240–6248

59. Matthews DA, Suchman AL, Branch WT (1993) Making connexions: enhancing the therapeutic potential of patient-clinician relationships." Ann Intern Med 118:973–977

60. Meier DE, Back AL, Morrison RS (2001) The inner life of physicians and care of the seriously ill. JAMA 268:3007–3014

61. Monge E, Sotomayor R (2004) Attitudes towards delivering bad news in Peru. Lancet 363:1556

62. Mook E, Chan F, Chan V et al. (2003) Family experience caring for terminally ill patients with cancer in Hong Kong. Cancer Nurs 26:267–275

63. Mystakidou K, Liossi CH, Vlachos L, Papadimitriou J (1996) Disclosure of diagnostic information to cancer patients in Greece. Palliat Med 10:195–200

64. Mystadikou K, Parpa E, Tsilika E at al. (2004) Cancer information disclosure in different cultural contexts. Supp Care Cancer 12:147–154

65. Nattinger AB (2005) Variation in the choice of breast-conserving surgery or mastectomy: patient or physician decision-making? J Clin Oncol 23:5429–5431

66. Nayak S, Pradhan JPB, Reddy S et al. (2005) Cancer patients' perceptions of the quality of communication before and after implementation of a communication strategy in a regional cancer center in India. J Clin Oncol 23:4771–4775

67. Nelson HL (1997) Stories and their limits. Narrative approaches to bioethics. Routledge, New York London

68. Newman J (1998) Managing cultural diversity: the art of communication. Radiol Technol 69:231–246

69. Novack DB, Plumer S, Smith RI et al. Changes in physicians' attidues toward telling the cancer patiant. JAMA 241:897–900

70. Olweny C (1994)The ethics and conduct of cross-cultural research in developing countries. Psycho-oncology 3:11–20

71. Oken D (1961) What to tell cancer patients. JAMA 175:1120–1128

72. Ozdogan M, Samur M, Bozcuk HS et al. (2004) "Do not tell": what factors affect relative' attitudes to honest disclosure of diagnosis to cancer patients? Supp Care Cancer 12:497–502

73. Parker PA, Baile WF, de Moor C et al. (2001) Breaking bad news about cancer: Patients' preferences for communication. J Clin Oncol 19:2049–2056

74. Pellegrino ED (1992) Is truth-telling to patients a cultural artifact? JAMA 268:1734–1735

75. Pellegrino ED, Thomasma DC.(1988) For the patient's good. The restoration of beneficence in health care. Oxford University Press, New York London

76. Phipps E, Ture G, Harris D et al. (2003) Approaching end of life : attitudes, preferences, and behaviors of African-American and White patients and their family care-givers. J Clin Oncol 21:549–554

77. Russell Searight H, Gafford J (2005) Cultural diversity at the end of life: issues and guidelines for family physicians. Am Fam Physician 71:515–522

78. Seibert PS, Stridh-Igo P, Zimmmermann CG (2002) A checklist to facilitate cultural awareness and sensitivity. J Med Ethics 28:143–146

79. Sekimoto M, Asai A, Ohnishi M et al. (2004) Patients' preferences for involvement in treatment decision making in Japan. BMC Fam Pract 5:1

80. Seo M, Tamura K, Shijo H et al. (2000) Telling the diagnosis to cancer patients in Japan: attitude and perceptions of patients, physicians and nurses. Palliat Med14:105–110

81. Sherwin S (1998) A relational approach to autonomy in health care. In: Sherwin S (ed) The Feminist Health Care Ethics Research Network. The politics of women's health: exploring agency and autonomy. Temple University Press, Philadelphia, pp 19–44

82. Spiro H (1993) What is empathy and can it be taught? In: Spiro H (ed) Empathy and the practice of medicine. Yale University Press, New Haven London

83. Spiro HM (2005) Tolling the truth. Part I. Science Med 18–23

84. Stewart M, Brown JB, Boon H et al. (1999) Evidence on patient-doctor communication. Cancer Prev Control 3:25–30

85. Surbone A (1992) Truth telling to the patient. JAMA 268:1661–1662

86. Surbone A (1993) The information to the cancer patient: psychosocial and spiritual implications. Supp Care Cancer 1:89–91

87. Surbone A (1997) Truth, risks and hope. Ann NY Acad Sci 809:73–80

88. Surbone A (2000a) The role of the family in the ethical dilemmas of oncology. In: Baider L, Cooper CL, De-Nour K (eds) Cancer and the family, 2nd edn. J. Wiley & Sons, Sussex, pp 513–534

89. Surbone A (2000b) Truth telling. Ann NY Acad Sci 913: 52–62

90. Surbone A (2003a) The quandary of cultural diversity. Guest editorial. J Pallliat Care 19:7–8

91. Surbone A (2003b) The difficult task of family care giving in oncology: exactly which roles do autonomy and gender play? Supp Care Cancer 11:617–619

92. Surbone A (2004a) Persisting differences in truth-telling throughout the world. Supp Care Cancer 12:143–146

93. Surbone A (2004b) Cultural competence: Why? Ann Oncol 15:697–699

94. Surbone A. (2005) Recognizing the patient as other. Supp Care Cancer 13:2–4

95. Surbone A, Lowenstein J (2003) Asymmetry in the patient-doctor relationship. J Clinic Ethics 14:183–188

96. Surbone A, Zwitter M (1997) Communication with the cancer patient: information and truth. Ann NY Acad Sci809

97. Surbone A, Ritossa C, Spagnolo AG (2004) Evolution of truth-telling attitudes and practices in Italy. Crit Rev Oncol Hematol 52:165–172

98. Swendson C, Windsor C (1996) Rethinking cultural diversity. Nurs Inquiry 3:3-10

99. Tse CY, Chong A, Fok SY (2003) Breaking bad news: a Chinese perspective. Palliat Medicine 17:339–343

100. Vega WA (2005) Higher stakes for cultural competence. Gen Hosp Psych 27:446–450

101. Voogt E, van Leeuwen AF, Visser AP et al. (2005) Information needs of patients with incurable cancer. Supp Care Cancer 13:943-948

102. Williams B (2002) Truth and truthfulness. An essay in genealogy. Princeton University Press, Princeton

103. Zweifler J, Gonzales AM (1998) Teaching residents to care for culturally diverse populations. Academic Med 73:1056–1061

10 Current Concepts of Communication Skills Training in Oncology

L. Fallowfield, V. Jenkins

© Springer-Verlag Berlin Heidelberg 2006

Summary

Too many patients leave their consultations with insufficient understanding about their diagnosis, prognosis, the need for further diagnostic tests, the management plans, or the therapeutic intent of treatment. This situation is not entirely due to paternalism or a lack of awareness that patients worldwide desire more information, but rather a reflection of the dismal communication skills training that most healthcare professionals receive. There have been many developments aimed at rectifying this situation, but there are still too few publications available demonstrating efficacy. Nevertheless, evidence shows that communication skills can be taught and that if taught well then the impact endures into the clinic. This chapter looks at some of the history of good evidence-based interventions to improve communication and makes a plea for more research-based evidence for improved patient outcomes following training. Unless attention and resources are given to help healthcare professionals in this core clinical skill then we will never be able to help patients and their families take an informed and educated role in their own cancer care.

"A successful dialogue between patient and physician is at the heart of working scientifically with patients."

George Engel, 1995

10.1 Short History

It is difficult to identify within the history of medicine when and in what form general communication skills training first began. It is probable that for centuries the old apprenticeship model pertained with students learning through observation of physicians on clinical ward rounds rather than from formal lectures or writings on the topic; certainly this was the primary method for all medical education in eighteenth century England. Back in the mid fifth century b.c., however, Hippocrates produced a code of ethics that included what doctors should do and say to comfort their patients (Lyons and Petrocelli 1978). We do not have a record of the exact form of words suggested, but we do know that Hippocrates' doctrine, unlike his contemporaries, emphasised the importance of the patient rather that the disease.

Not until 1927 did Francis Peabody (Peabody 1984), a clinician working in Boston USA, focus the spotlight back on communication between the clinician and the patient. In this landmark article "The Secret to the Care of the Patient", he noted that the most common criticism made by older practitioners was that young graduates "are too 'scientific' and do not know how to take care of patients." What Dr. Peabody voiced almost 80 years ago was that medicine focussed on the biology of disease and ignored important psychosocial factors and effective communication that were essential to the development of a good physician–patient relationship.

In the 1960s the interview became the focus of research, and evidence emerged demonstrating that health professionals really needed to be taught effective communication skills. Many clinicians believed that you either possessed these skills or not, and that no amount of teaching would change people's behaviours. Some of the earliest (now seminal) studies published emphasising the need for communication skills training came from the work of Barbara Korsch and Vida Negrete, who observed doctor–parent communication within a large paediatric clinic (Korsch and Negrete 1972). The study involved videotaping interactions between doctors and parents of sick infants followed by immediate and delayed interviews. These interviews examined parents' satisfaction with the doctor's performance, their understanding of the terminology used in the consultations and how much the parents complied with the doctor's instructions. The detailed findings from over 800 cases highlighted barriers to effective communication, specifically doctors' use of technical language, not addressing the parents' concerns directly, and being too business-like in their approach. The results also identified evidence of good communication skills and showed that when the parent had an active interaction with the doctor, compliance with treatment and satisfaction were higher.

Communication skills training for medicine developed in earnest around the time of this influential work, and George Engel in the United States pioneered his patient-centred approaches when teaching medical interviewing, which will be described later. Although primary care physicians early on embraced the need for patient-centred interactions through better communication, specific training targeted at the healthcare professionals working in oncology only really began in the late 1980s. This setting has been the focus for considerable research around the development and evaluation of communication skills training in the past 20 years.

10.2   Why CST Training: Background

"The chief virtue that language can have is clearness, and nothing detracts from it so much as the use of unfamiliar words."

Hippocrates

Although the essentials of effective communication remain the same whatever the setting, consultations about cancer contain many difficulties. The specific problems and situations encountered need elaboration and also research to enable a core teaching programme with relevant and evidence-based content. Too often the communication skills courses available are generic in focus and fail to define precisely the content and context in which specific skills are most likely to enhance the interaction. Moreover, much of the early research about doctor–patient communication arose from primary care settings; many of these interviews, where patients may arrive with a plethora of psychosocial and psychosomatic concerns, differ substantially from those within oncology. An anxious patient with a personal or social problem that manifests itself through complaints about headaches and sleep difficulties may need a very different interaction with her doctor than one anxious to receive the results of the scan that reveals a cerebral tumour. Although patients being investigated for cancer would welcome some psychosocial enquiry and identification of their concerns, arguably they might be more interested in learning the nature of their disease and importantly the treatment. Using a typical primary care interview as a template for communication skills training might not be appropriate in an oncology setting where information giving is vital and likely to result in the doctor speaking more than the patient. Learning how to pace complex information and provide it in a flexible manner appropriate for patients with different educational, social and cultural backgrounds, whilst being empathic and responding to patient-led cues is not easy in a busy clinic, and healthcare professionals receive little training in this core clinical skill. For those involved in teaching, a clear understanding of

Table 1 The DREAM interview: key components and skills needed

Data	Collecting accurate data, e.g. taking a clear medical history of needs knowledge about appropriate use of open, focused open and closed questions and avoidance of leading and multiple questions
Relationship	Establishing a relationship or rapport, e.g. learning more about patient's worries and concerns and making patient feel comfortable by giving and asking information; not interrupting too much or looking at notes; needs awareness of verbal and non-verbal communication and ability to engage in active listening
Empathy	Being empathic, e.g. responding to appropriately to patient-led cues; acknowledging burden of disease and treatment
Advice	Giving advice, e.g. explaining logic and rationale for treatment; putting complex information into layman's terms; needs ability to structure information giving into manageable chunks, to summarise and constantly check understanding
Motivation	Providing motivation, e.g. ensuring that patient understands the true therapeutic intent of treatment and feels motivated to embark on therapy with likelihood of achieving realistic goals; needs unambiguous use of language; ability to focus patient on goals such as improving quality of life

the structure of the interview together with acknowledgement of some of the likely barriers to effective communication is paramount.

Some of the communication difficulties found in typical oncology consultations may include breaking bad news about diagnosis or recurrence, giving results or describing the need for further diagnostic tests, explaining complex treatment options and clinical trials, obtaining informed consent and discussing transitions from active therapy to palliative care (Fallowfield and Jenkins 1999). All these potential topics need to be set against a framework for the interaction which has been described as the DREAM interview. See Table 1.

10.3 Results of Poor Communication in Cancer

Unless a doctor can find some way of understanding how a patient integrates and then interprets the often quite complex biomedical information into his everyday world and experiences, the dialogue between them largely proceeds as two parallel and separate monologues. The specifics and detail in explanations about diagnostic tests and management plans and an affective appreciation for the life context within which the

patient places these, are necessary prerequisites for successful and effective communication between patients and their doctors.

Poor communication can result in faulty clinical data collection, worsened clinical and psychosocial outcomes, greater likelihood of litigation (Levinson et al. 1997) and confusion over prognosis (Hagerty et al. 2005). In addition, many patients feel that they have received insufficient information and have not been properly involved in decision making about their treatment and care (Davison et al. 1995; Degner et al. 1997). A recent study examined the relationships between decisional role (preferred and assumed) at time of surgical treatment (baseline), congruence between assumed role at baseline and preferred role 3 years later (follow-up), and quality of life in 205 women diagnosed with breast cancer (Hack et al. 2005). The authors reported that a statistically significant number of women had decisional role regret, with most preferring greater involvement in treatment planning than was offered. Women who indicated at baseline that they were actively involved in choosing their surgical treatment had significantly higher overall quality of life at follow-up than women who indicated passive involvement. These actively involved women had significantly higher physical and social functioning and significantly less fatigue than women who assumed a passive role.

In another study involving women with breast cancer, benefits accrued to women being treated by doctors who offered choice of surgery wherever possible (Fallowfield et al. 1994). The results had little to do with choice, however, as even women who could not exercise choice due to constraints such as tumour size had reduced levels of psychological morbidity. The reason for this finding was that doctors who tried to involve patients as much as possible were better communicators and provided much more information about the rationale for treatments being suggested.

Patients today are more aware than ever of what to expect and the sorts of treatments available, which they may have read about through the media or on the Internet. This can either be a help or hindrance to a consultation, depending on whether the patient is well informed or misinformed. Also, there are different types of consultations that require their own complex language, for example discussing treatment options with patients as part of randomised clinical trials (Jenkins et al. 2005).

Most healthcare professionals working within the cancer setting experience some emotional reaction and degree of job dissatisfaction during their career. This can be a reaction to the pressure from management to increase the speed with which patients are diagnosed and treated, often without additional resources and infrastructure. Problematic communication with patients is thought to contribute to emotional burnout and low personal accomplishment (job satisfaction) as well as high psychological morbidity in clinicians (Ramirez et al. 1996), and this finding has not changed perceptibly in 10 years (Taylor et al. 2005). Ramirez and colleagues reported that doctors acknowledged that poor communication and management skills training contributed to their psychological distress and burnout.

Ineffective communication also has negative effects on patient care and causes stress when nurses interact with each other, medical colleagues, patients and relatives (Fallowfield et al. 2001b). As much of the delivery of healthcare services is handled by multidisciplinary teams (Jenkins et al. 2001; Catt et al. 2005), communication between and within teams must be clear and unambiguous to help avoid errors and to

ensure that accountability for system failures is recognised and acted upon (Firth-Cozens 2001).

A recent (2002) report by the independent National Confidential Enquiry into Perioperative Deaths (www.ncepod.org.uk/) cited poor communication and teamwork as major contributory factors in the large numbers of deaths that occur within 3 days of a medical intervention. There is some evidence that traditional hierarchical barriers and differing perceptions of informational roles in healthcare teams make discussion about errors problematic (Sexton et al. 2000). The likelihood that errors will be accurately reported and identified so that individuals and systems can benefit and protect future patients may be less in dysfunctional teams.

Many malpractice complaints stem from poor communication vs negligence or error (Vincent et al. 1994). In the US particularly, litigation is a major concern costing billions of dollars annually. There is evidence that sued and non-sued physicians have different styles of communication (Levinson et al. 1997) and that major insurance agencies provide discounts to doctors who attend communications skills training courses.

10.4 Different Ways of Teaching CST

"Learners respond best to the same values as patients do—caring, respect, understanding, empathy and competence."

Lipkin 1995

Communication skills training should bring benefits to both the patient and the health professional. It is widely accepted that communication skills need to be taught and that even senior professionals can acquire new skills that translate into the clinical setting and are enduring (Fallowfield et al. 2002, 2003). Despite the existence of level 1 evidence that communication skills training improves the way health professionals interact with patients, there are no clear guidelines about what form of training to use. Many different approaches have been taken by educators attempting to improve communication skills of healthcare professionals within oncology. One of the most influential models for teaching communication skills to groups of physicians was developed by Mack Lipkin. The Lipkin model itself drew on the contributions from psychiatrists George Engel and Carl Rogers, together with the educational theories of Knowles (1980) and Friere (1986). Fallowfield and colleagues modified this original Lipkin model for use within oncology (Fallowfield et al. 1998).

These types of residential courses are learner-centred, incorporating cognitive, affective and behavioural components. Participants work in small groups of 3–5 individuals, led by an experienced facilitator and role-play with patient simulators (actors) skilled in providing constructive feedback from role-playing. In these types of communication skills training courses, each clinician/health professional identifies the communication problems most important to him and then works on ways of resolving at least one of these through role-play with patient simulators followed by video review and group discussion. Training courses based on this model are rated highly by participants (Fallowfield et al. 2001b, 2002) and although resource intensive, they do result in beneficial changes in communication behaviours that translate into the clinical setting and are enduring (Fallowfield et al. 2003).

In a recent systematic review of communication training methods for health professionals who work with patients with cancer, only four were grade 1a randomised controlled trials (Gysels et al. 2005). These were the work of Klein et al. (1999), Fallowfield et al. (2002), and two by Darius Razavi's group in Belgium (Razavi et al. 1993, 2002). Klein and colleagues focussed on the effects of using patients with cancer in teaching communication skills to 233 medical undergraduates, and the investigators re-evaluated 54 of these students 2 years later. Students were randomised to be taught communication skills either with patients who had cancer or patients with other illnesses. The study took place within an interview methods course for third-year medical students, and two outcome measures were used to assess their performance. One examined attitudes of students towards what they consider to be important characteristics of hospital doctors and attitudes towards various aspects of the management of patients. The other rated a video

recording of the students interviewing a real patient. The authors reported that the experimental group had better ratings in terms of responding empathically, showing regard and concern for the patient and assessing the impact of the symptoms on a patient's life. Razavi's work with oncology nurses focussed on a variety of skills as a component of a more psychological training package. The first study looked at the effects that a 24-h psychological training programme had on the attitudes, communication skills and occupational stress in oncology nurses. The nurses were randomised to attend training courses (eight weekly sessions of 3 h) or a waiting list. Communication skills were assessed via videotaped role-play with simulated patients. In this study, limited changes were found in communication behaviours; the only significant change that occurred was that the intervention group was more "in control" of the interview (Razavi et al. 1993). In their later study, the nurses were videotaped under two conditions, a simulated interview with an actor and a clinical interview with a cancer patient. They reported an increase in emotionally laden words used by those nurses who had attended training compared to those in the control group, and this increase in emotional word use facilitated patients' expressions of emotion (Razavi et al. 2002).

A similar finding of improved communication in nurses occurred in two studies by Wilkinson and colleagues; their participants followed less-intensive training programs but ones that still retained role-play with feedback (3-day residential and non-residential courses; Wilkinson et al. 2002, 2003). However it is important to note that several studies found in the literature focus on improving participants' ability to assess psychological and emotional well-being rather than to improve communication in the more extensive topics required in an oncology clinic by a clinician.

Role-play accompanied by constructive feedback in a safe environment appears to be one of the key factors in changing communication behaviours. Yet often it causes anxiety for many health professionals because they have had previous encounters that were unsatisfactory. This particularly concerns those courses or workshops involving group members taking turns to "play the patient" or those run by inexperienced facilitators who do not set up appropriate scenarios, with clearly defined goals and objectives and who are cognizant of all the safety rules that must be observed when running such sessions. More credible role-play—that is videotaped and then reviewed via feedback led by an experienced facilitator and simulated patient—has been shown to be an excellent medium to raise a medical student's awareness of the range of potential communication challenges they could encounter throughout their clinical career (Nestel and Kidd 2002; Nestel et al. 2002). Trained actors who work as patient simulators provide a safe opportunity for healthcare staff to practice different communication behaviours without distressing patients (Razavi et al. 2000).

10.5   What Can Be Improved?

Stewart's review of studies examining effective doctor–patient communication and patient health outcomes cites only four with level 1 evidence of significant patient benefits (Stewart 1995). These involved (1) doctors in general practice in Australia who attended 3-h seminars on patient history-taking (Evans et al. 1987), (2) clinicians who either received 8-h training in verbal skills to handle emotion or verbal skills for problem solving or no intervention (Bertakis et al. 1991) (3) and those that involved interventions to increase patient involvement in consultations (Greenfield et al. 1988; Kaplan et al. 1989). The types of health outcomes measured across the studies included anxiety levels, distress, blood pressure, blood glucose levels, functional status and patient satisfaction. Although none of the studies specifically involved oncology patients and clinicians, the significant improvement in patient health outcomes would suggest that effective communication has a positive influence on patients' health.

However, research on patient outcomes following communication skills training for cancer consultations has been limited. In a review of different training programs to improve communication for health professionals who care for cancer patients, few of the studies mention pa-

tient outcomes (Gysels et al. 2004). Fallowfield and colleagues examined patient satisfaction and clinicians' ability to detect distress in patients following communication skills training (Fallowfield et al. 2001a; Shilling et al. 2003). The overall score for patient satisfaction was related to patient's age, level of psychological morbidity and, most significantly, with the length of wait time in the clinic. There was a tendency for greater satisfaction for patients of doctors who had attended the course that was not present in patients of doctors with no intervention.

More recent work has focussed on providing interventions for patients with the goal of improving the doctor–patient dialogue. One such study has a measure of quality of life as the patient outcome (Velikova et al. 2004), and although it is not an outcome following communication skills training course , it is an outcome that could be employed in future studies.

10.6   Future of CST

The case for serious communications skills training for all healthcare professionals has been made for several years now, and many higher education institutions have responded by including more of this in the curriculum for nurses, doctors and other professions allied to medicine. The methods of training are not always appropriate, however, with far too much reliance on telling students the 'right' and 'wrong' ways of communicating via didactic lectures, passive observation or large group discussion. Few of these methods are likely to help students develop the flexible and challenging skills needed to help their patients and to provide satisfying and professionally and personally rewarding interactions. Nor should communication skills training be exclusively part of the psychiatry or primary care rotations and taught solely therefore by practitioners in those disciplines aided by the odd psychologist or social worker. Arguably the most credible role-models for trainees are their senior colleagues, and so we need to continue to conduct advanced communication skills programmes for experienced healthcare professionals as well. There is little point in equipping junior staff in better skills if they then enter the same old system that has consummately failed to provide excellent communicators. There is a continuing need for top-down as well as bottom-up training so that juniors have good role-models to emulate, and their own endeavours to improve and develop well-rounded communication skills are encouraged and rewarded.

In the UK—as part of the 2000 Cancer Plan (UK Department of Health 2000) supported centrally by government—an ambitious programme has started whereby a cadre of healthcare professionals are being trained as facilitators to run 3-day residential courses for doctors, nurses and other multi-professional groups in oncology. The model is consistent and based on evidence for efficacy, and all facilitators have to pass specific competencies before being funded to run courses for colleagues. Such programmes are resource-intensive but necessary if we are genuinely to improve the skills base for the benefit of all—healthcare professional and patient.

References

1. Bertakis KD, Roter D, Putnam SM (1991) The relationship of physician medical interview style to patient satisfaction. J Fam Pract 32:175–181
2. Catt S, Fallowfield L, Jenkins V, Langridge C, Cox A (2005) The informational roles and psychological health of members of 10 oncology multidisciplinary teams in the UK. Br J Cancer 93:1092–1097
3. Davison BJ, Degner LF, Morgan TR (1995) Information and decision-making preferences of men with prostate cancer. Oncol Nurs Forum 22:1401–1408
4. Degner LF, Kristjanson LJ, Bowman D, Sloan JA, Carriere KC, O'Neil J, Bilodeau B, Watson P, Mueller B (1997) Information needs and decisional preferences in women with breast cancer. JAMA 277:1485–1492
5. Evans BJ, Kiellerup FD, Stanley RO, Burrows GD, Sweet B (1987) A communication skills programme for increasing patients' satisfaction with general practice consultations. Br J Med Psychol 60:373–378
6. Fallowfield L, Jenkins V (1999) Effective communication skills are the key to good cancer care. Eur J Cancer 35:1592–1597
7. Fallowfield L, Lipkin M, Hall A (1998) Teaching senior oncologists communication skills: results from phase I of a comprehensive longitudinal program in the United Kingdom. J Clin Oncol 16:1961–1968
8. Fallowfield L, Ratcliffe D, Jenkins V, Saul J (2001a) Psychiatric morbidity and its recognition by doctors in patients with cancer. Br J Cancer 84:1011–1015
9. Fallowfield L, Saul J, Gilligan B (2001b) Teaching senior nurses how to teach communication skills in oncology. Cancer Nurs 24:185–191
10. Fallowfield L, Jenkins V, Farewell V, Saul J, Duffy A, Eves R (2002) Efficacy of a Cancer Research UK communication skills training model for oncologists: a randomised controlled trial. Lancet 359:650–656
11. Fallowfield L, Jenkins V, Farewell V, Solis-Trapala I (2003) Enduring impact of communication skills training: results of a 12-month follow-up. Br J Cancer 89:1445–1449
12. Fallowfield LJ, Hall A, Maguire P, Baum M, A'Hern RP (1994) Psychological effects of being offered choice of surgery for breast cancer. BMJ 309:448
13. Firth-Cozens J (2001) Multidisciplinary teamwork: the good, bad, and everything in between. Qual Health Care 10:65–66
14. Greenfield S, Kaplan SH, Ware JE Jr, Yano EM, Frank HJ (1988) Patients' participation in medical care: effects on blood sugar control and quality of life in diabetes. J Gen Intern Med 3:448–457
15. Gysels M, Richardson A, Higginson IJ (2004) Communication training for health professionals who care for patients with cancer: a systematic review of effectiveness. Support Care Cancer 12:692–700
16. Gysels M, Richardson A, Higginson IJ (2005) Communication training for health professionals who care for patients with cancer: a systematic review of training methods. Support Care Cancer 13:356–366
17. Hack TF, Degner LF, Watson P, Sinha L (2005) Do patients benefit from participating in medical decision making? Longitudinal follow-up of women with breast cancer. Psychooncology 15:9–19
18. Hagerty RG, Butow PN, Ellis PM, Dimitry S, Tattersall MH (2005) Communicating prognosis in cancer care: a systematic review of the literature. Ann Oncol 16:1005–1053

19. Jenkins V, Fallowfield L, Solis-Trapala I, Langridge C, Farewell V (2005) Discussing randomised clinical trials of cancer therapy: evaluation of a Cancer Research UK training programme. BMJ 330:400

20. Jenkins VA, Fallowfield LJ, Poole K (2001) Are members of multidisciplinary teams in breast cancer aware of each other's informational roles? Qual Health Care 10:70–75

21. Kaplan SH, Greenfield S, Ware JE Jr (1989) Assessing the effects of physician-patient interactions on the outcomes of chronic disease. Med Care 27:S110–S127

22. Klein S, Tracy D, Kitchener HC, Walker LG (1999) The effects of the participation of patients with cancer in teaching communication skills to medical undergraduates: a randomised study with follow-up after 2 years. Eur J Cancer 35:1448–1456

23. Korsch BM, Negrete VF (1972) Doctor-patient communication. Sci Am 227:66–74

24. Levinson W, Roter DL, Mullooly JP, Dull VT, Frankel RM (1997) Physician-patient communication. The relationship with malpractice claims among primary care physicians and surgeons. JAMA 277:553–559

25. Lyons AS, Petrocelli RJ (1978) Medicine: an illustrated history. Abradale Press, New York

26. Nestel D, Kidd J (2002) Evaluating a teaching skills workshop for medical students. Med Educ 36:1094–1095

27. Nestel D, Muir E, Plant M, Kidd J, Thurlow S (2002) Modelling the lay expert for first-year medical students: the actor-patient as teacher. Med Teach 24:562–564

28. Peabody FW (1984) Landmark article March 19, 1927: the care of the patient. By Francis W. Peabody. JAMA 252:813–818

29. Ramirez AJ, Graham J, Richards MA, Timothy AR (1996) Stress at work for the clinical oncologist. Clin Oncol 8:137–139

30. Razavi D, Delvaux N, Marchal S, Bredart A, Farvacques C, Paesmans M (1993) The effects of a 24-h psychological training program on attitudes, communication skills and occupational stress in oncology: a randomised study. Eur J Cancer 29A:1858–1863

31. Razavi D, Delvaux N, Marchal S, De Cock M, Farvacques C, Slachmuylder JL (2000) Testing health care professionals' communication skills: the usefulness of highly emotional standardized role-playing sessions with simulators. Psychooncology 9:293–302

32. Razavi D, Delvaux N, Marchal S, Durieux JF, Farvacques C, Dubus L, Hogenraad R (2002) Does training increase the use of more emotionally laden words by nurses when talking with cancer patients? A randomised study. Br J Cancer 87:1–7

33. Sexton JB, Thomas EJ, Helmreich RL (2000) Error, stress and teamwork in medicine and aviation. A cross-sectional study. Chirurg 71:suppl 138–142

34. Shilling V, Jenkins V, Fallowfield L (2003) Factors affecting patient and clinician satisfaction with the clinical consultation: can communication skills training for clinicians improve satisfaction? Psychooncology 12:599–611

35. Stewart MA (1995) Effective physician-patient communication and health outcomes: a review. CMAJ 152:1423–1433

36. Taylor C, Graham J, Potts HW, Richards MA, Ramirez AJ (2005) Changes in mental health of UK hospital consultants since the mid-1990s. Lancet 366:742–744

37. UK Department of Health (2000) The NHS cancer plan: a plan for investment, a plan for reform. NHS, London

38. Velikova G, Booth L, Smith AB, Brown PM, Lynch P, Brown JM, Selby PJ (2004) Measuring quality of life in routine oncology practice improves communication and patient well-being: a randomized controlled trial. J Clin Oncol 22:714–724

39. Vincent C, Young M, Phillips A (1994) Why do people sue doctors? A study of patients and relatives taking legal action. Lancet 343:1609–1613

40. Wilkinson SM, Gambles M, Roberts A (2002) The essence of cancer care: the impact of training on nurses' ability to communicate effectively. J Adv Nurs 40:731–738

41. Wilkinson SM, Leliopoulou C, Gambles M, Roberts A (2003) Can intensive three-day programmes improve nurses' communication skills in cancer care? Psychooncology 12:747–759

11 Communication Skills Training in Oncology: It Works!

F. Stiefel, N. Favre, J.N. Despland

Recent Results in Cancer Research, Vol. 168
© Springer-Verlag Berlin Heidelberg 2006

Summary

While the previous chapter by L. Fallowfield and V. Jenkins focuses on different communication skills training (CST) concepts currently being utilized, this chapter reviews and comments the scientific evidence of the impact of CST on improving communication skills. The aim of this chapter is not to provide a complete review of the evidence—this has already been done in systematic reviews—but to discuss the scientific evidence and reflect on the available results and relevant topics for further investigations.

11.1 Rationale for CST in Oncology

Communication skills training (CST) is based on the assumptions that (1) communication with patients requires specific skills, (2) these skills are relevant, and (3) such skills can be improved by training.

Communication with patients is not restricted to providing medical information. A medical consultation consists of cognitive, emotional, and relational aspects and requires specific skills, especially in oncology, since complex information is provided and vital decisions have to be made (Ong et al. 1995, 2000). Important differences with regard to communication skills have been observed among oncology clinicians: For example, some clinicians utilize avoidance strategies, such as denial of patients' emotional suffering by focusing on medical information only; others respond empathically to the patients' cues and also discuss emotional and social aspects of disease (Guex et al. 2002; Wilkinson 1991). The important communicational variability observed, one can assume—and this has been confirmed by scientific and clinical observations—that specific communication skills are required in clinical practice (Fallowfield et al. 1998).

The relevance of communication in oncology has also been confirmed: Poor communication increases a patient's psychological distress (Ford et al. 1996; Lerman et al. 1993; Razavi et al. 2000) and hampers his quality of life, adjustment to illness, and adherence to treatment (Razavi et al. 2000), and may lead to dissatisfaction and increased risk of litigation (Ford et al. 1996; Loge et al. 1997). In addition, poor communication also has a negative impact on stress of the medical staff and increases burnout (Fallowfield 1995; Ramirez et al. 1996).

Finally, effective communication skills are not just inborn qualities or a simple by-product of the professional experience (Fallowfield et al. 1998; Maguire et al. 1996); it has been shown that they can be modified and improved by specific training programs (Fallowfield et al. 1998, 2002, 2003; Gysels et al. 2004; Jenkins and Fallowfield 2002; Maguire et al. 1996).

CST is time-consuming and costly; it requires a high degree of motivation and induces a considerable stress in participants, since CST uses techniques that are confronting, such as feedback to participants about their videotaped interviews with (simulated) patients. Since communication is a central element in oncology, such an effort is justified as long as this training proves to be effective. A meaningful scientific investigation of CST is therefore necessary. Such research is challenging, yet not impossible to realize. The following paragraphs aim to discuss the results and limitations of current research on CST in oncology.

11.2 Objectives and Setting of CST

Different forms of CST have been developed, addressing different populations such as medical students (Klein 1999), transplantation specialists who deal with sensitive issues like organ donation (Fitzgerald et al. 2004), or oncology clinicians (Fallowfield et al. 1998, 2003; Jenkins and Fallowfield 2002; Wilkinson et al. 2002). In Switzerland, CST has become mandatory for physicians who wish to specialize in oncology (Hürny 2000). The objectives of CST are shaped by the professional and cultural background of the trainers and participants. Some trainings focus on breaking bad news, others on patient needs assessment, empathic response, or relational aspects of communication (Gysels et al. 2005). Most often, different objectives co-exist and many of them are interrelated. For example, to respond with empathy to a patient's distress is only possible if the relational aspects of a consultation are perceived, if the patient's needs are acknowledged, and if the understanding of the situation includes the psychological aspects. And a clinician who responds empathically will also deliver bad news in a way that makes the patient feel contained and understood. Nevertheless, to define specific objectives of CST is important, especially for educational purposes; however, in clinical reality, these objectives cannot be separated, since they are part of a whole.

With regards to participants, CST most often addresses nurses and physicians; some are mono-disciplinary and others interdisciplinary, and the number of participants varies considerably (Gysels et al. 2005). Interdisciplinary training has the advantage of increasing mutual understanding between members of the medical staff—misunderstandings being a common source of confu-

sion and mismanagement with a negative impact on the patient. As long as the number of nurses and physicians is balanced, interdisciplinary training seems to have a clear advantage. In some cultural contexts, however, it may be that physicians are still reluctant to work on such sensitive issues together with nurses. We have found that nurses often respond more adequate to patients' distress than physicians, while the latter often have a greater ability to structure the consultation. No study has yet addressed the question of whether a mono- or interdisciplinary approach produces different outcomes. The number of participants is also a crucial variable. We work with small groups of 8–10 participants; and feedback on videotaped interviews with simulated patients is provided in subgroups of 4 participants (Favre et al. 2006). One can easily imagine that this setting allows for a much more secure and individualized atmosphere than training programs with larger groups. In studies evaluating CST in oncology, groups ranged from 3 to 40 participants (Gysels et al. 2005). The literature still lacks data on cost-effectiveness of CST with regard to the number of participants.

Professional backgrounds of teachers and teaching methods also differ. CST teachers in oncology are usually psychiatrists or psychologists. While the above-mentioned systematic review did not identify the professional background and qualification of teachers, we firmly believe that only experienced psychiatrists or psychologists working in consultation-liaison psychiatry or psycho-oncology should provide such training. The key to success for many participants involves being confronted with their communicational difficulties in a way that respects their narcissistic vulnerability. The credibility of the teachers depends on their capacity to build a constructive and safe atmosphere, to react adequately to group phenomena, to manage "difficult" participants and their profound knowledge of the professional environment of the participants.

Duration of CST is another factor influencing outcome. Training sessions evaluated scientifically (Gysels et al. 2005) were either provided in workshops of a few days duration or in sessions spread over a period of a few weeks; there is certainly a time limit below which the effect of a CST will not be satisfactory. The benefits of booster sessions, for example, have been demonstrated (Razavi et al. 2003).

The fact that there are various types of CST, which differ with regard to objectives, duration, number and professional background of participants, and qualification of teachers, does not facilitate their scientific evaluation. The level of evidence of their evaluation varies, with only 13 studies (out of 47) meeting the inclusion criteria of a systematic review (Gysels et al. 2005): Only four were grade 1a randomized controlled trials; most of the other studies were based on a single-group pre/post test design.

11.3 CST: What Works?

Most CST in oncology utilizes an interactive approach focusing on role-play, feedback to videotaped or audiotaped interviews with simulated patients, and small-group discussions of case presentations. The training usually lasts several days, sometimes followed by individual supervision and booster sessions.

The heterogeneity of CST is problematic from a scientific point of view. It is difficult to compare the studies or include them in a meta-analysis. From a clinical point of view, however, standardization is counterproductive and hampers learner-centered methods, most effective in postgraduate education. CST seems to be effective if individualized and if the training corresponds to the clinical reality. What is a difficulty from the scientific point of view is therefore a necessity from an educational point of view and should not lead to the wrong conclusion that studies of CST are less "scientific" or that only CST utilizing highly standardized, evidenced-based approaches should be implemented. On the contrary, such CST may be inappropriate, since they neither reflect real world conditions, nor are they participant-centered.

Another problem with the studies investigating CST concerns the fact that a CST session has various effective elements. This may be illustrated by a few examples based on views of these training methods from different psychological perspectives. Participants learn new ways

of communication by means of case discussions, role-playing, and feedback to videotaped interviews. From a cognitive point of view, one may argue that case discussions modify the mental representation of how to interact with patients and introduces a broader set of possible responses and thus a more patient-centered approach. From a behavioral point of view, one may argue that role-playing enables participants to experience new ways of communicating and thus a more patient-centered approach. From a psychodynamic point of view, one may argue that feedback increases self-awareness of the participants' own communication style, identification with experienced teachers and peers, a growing understanding of relational aspects, and thus a more patient-centered approach.

While from a scientific point of view the coexistence of different "active" elements makes it difficult to understand how CST works, from an educational point of view it is well known that only training based on different didactic approaches combining theoretical knowledge with practical exercises is effective. Methods based on a unique didactic approach are condemned to fail, since participants have different learning styles and benefit from various educational components. What seems problematic from a scientific point of view is therefore a necessity from an educational point of view.

11.4 CST in Oncology: Outcomes

Different outcomes of CST have been identified: (1) behavioral assessment, (2) patient outcomes, and (3) participants' self report. Behavioral assessment is based on coding of various aspects of communication, such as speaking time of the simulated patient, interruptions by the physician, or number of open questions. The aim of behavioral assessments is to evaluate if patient-centered communication can be improved. Patient-outcome studies evaluate the impact of CST on the patient; they are based on patients' judgment (e.g., satisfaction, comments, or feelings). Self-report studies rate the perceived change of participants (skills, ability to apply new skills, or confidence in communication). These three different outcome measurements have been utilized alone or in combination. All of them have advantages and disadvantages.

In behavioral assessment, video- or audio-taped interviews with simulated or "real" patients are coded and scored by trained and independent raters using standardized methods (Booth and Maguire 1991; Ford et al. 2000; Roter 2002; Wilkinson 1991). While this method produces statistically meaningful categories of desired and undesired training effects, thus reflecting a certain objectivity, this approach may also be problematic. Some aspects of communication that are not coded by these methods will not be analyzed; for example, nuances and non-verbal signs, which provide meaning and foster therapeutic alliance, are omitted in the evaluation process. In addition, even if a given behavior falls into a "positive" category of the rating system, it may not be adequate in specific medical situations: For example, if a patient is anxious and overwhelmed, it might not be adequate to challenge him with open questions and to focus on his emotions; instead, it would be more appropriate to provide relevant information and guidance.

Patient outcomes, the second category of measurements utilized (Faulkner et al. 1995; Heaven and Maguire 1996), evaluate the direct impact of training on the patient. This seems, at first glance, the most elegant method to evaluate CST, since their ultimate objective is to improve communication with the patient. While this approach may be clinically meaningful, it is difficult to realize from a methodological point of view. In a pre/post design, different patients or different clinical situations have to be evaluated. If different patients are included, the impact of the training may be biased by patient selection. If the same patients are included, the clinical situations have evolved, presenting different challenges for the patient and the clinician; in addition, a most important variable of communication, the physician–patient relationship, has been fostered and thus a beneficial outcome may be its direct consequence. Randomized clinical trials, on the other hand, include different clinicians, different clinical situations, and different patients, all of which represent important confounding variables and imply that a high number of subjects have to be included in a study.

Finally, participants' self reports on changing attitudes (Fallowfield et al. 1998; Jenkins and Fallowfield 2002; Klein 1999) are measured. However, increased awareness does not imply a change in clinical practice. Participants' self reports may be influenced by the participants' social desirability and their need to show that their efforts were beneficial. One interesting approach is based on the participants' capacity of self-criticism when reviewing their interaction with a patient (Wilkinson et al. 1998, 1999, 2002), which may reflect an increased awareness when interacting with patients. Again, this approach does not provide evidence that communication really improves, and clinicians who are generally self-critical may bias the results.

Another important question is whether a benefit of CST is maintained over time. For example, the Swiss model (Hürny 2000) provides each oncology clinician with individual supervision 4–6 times over 6 months after the initial CST of 2 days. These sessions are utilized by participants in various ways. Some participants present recurrent difficulties with patients; others discuss emotionally charged situations. A few elaborate on their own psychological difficulties, which sometimes lead them to initiate psychological treatment. From our point of view, these individual sessions certainly help to induce change. There is a lack of studies evaluating the benefits of follow-up and booster sessions and the long-term effect of CST.

Taking into account the difficulties associated with the scientific evaluation of CST, a systemic review (Gysels et al. 2005) concluded that studies based on behavioral assessment achieved positive outcomes for different parameters such as open questions, empathy, responses to patients cues, control of the interview, and exploration of patients' feelings. Studies assessing patient outcomes failed to demonstrate an effect. Studies based on physician's self rating showed changes of attitudes, an increased sense of responsibility when telling bad news, improved confidence and satisfaction, as well as enhanced self-criticism when listening to audiotapes of consultations. Some of these studies showed maintenance of improvement after several months, others only reported post-training improvements but not long-lasting effects.

11.5 CST: How Does It Work?

One of the unanswered questions regarding CST is how improvement is achieved. Up to now, studies only addressed the question of whether CST had an impact or not. However, as with any other intervention, it is also important to understand how such training induces change.

Probably one of the most powerful variables of variance in outcome is the participant himself. We observe that some participants show an impressive increase in their communicational flexibility, leading to skilled patient-centered consultations, while others seem not to benefit from CST.

An understanding of how CST works may lead to the conceptualization of more specific training sessions, focusing on elements of communicational progress. If one considers CST as a psychological intervention with an educational objective, one wonders why such training includes professionals without restrictions. For any other psychological intervention, indication is an important issue. For example, behavioral interventions may be most effective for some clinical problems such as phobic behavior, but they are not suitable for persons who wish to understand how biographical circumstances influence their ways of relating to others. Since CST sessions are psychological interventions aimed at inducing change in the interactions participants have with their patients, inclusion criteria are important.

A brief case report from one of the communication skills seminars conducted in Switzerland illustrates this point.

Upon reviewing his videotaped interview with a simulated patient, a 38-year-old male physician suddenly cried out, "It's not me, it's my dead brother on the tape," broke into tears and ran out of the room. After a brief discussion with one of the teachers, he returned back to the session and was motivated and able to continue to review a short part of the video without misinterpretations.

The distress of the situation and the painful remembrance of his brother's death induced in this vulnerable man a brief psychotic episode. This example illustrates that CST can have negative impacts and that inclusion of participants should be based on an indication, as with other psychological interventions. Before defining indications and inclusion criteria, we should understand how CST works.

11.6 Psychodynamic Hypotheses Concerning CST

None of the published studies has addressed the question of how CST induces change. We will therefore present some preliminary results of a current study of our group addressing this issue. The aim of this paragraph is not to discuss methodological aspects of this project, but to illustrate a possible scientific approach.

Our interest focuses on the question of how oncology clinicians handle emotionally charged consultations. According to the psychodynamic approach, an individual faces distressing emotions by mobilizing defense mechanisms, which serve to protect him. We hypothesized that emotionally charged consultations trigger clinicians' defense mechanisms, which are more or less adaptive; if not adapted, they may hamper communication, empathy, and recognition of patients' suffering. Our main hypothesis is that CST modifies defense mechanisms of participants, leading to a more adaptative, patient-centered communication style. In a pilot study, verbatim transcriptions of videotaped interviews with simulated patients were evaluated before (n=10) and after CST (n=10) with the Defense Mechanism Rating Scales (DMRS) (Perry and Cooper 1989 ; Perry 1990). A wide variety of defense mechanisms were observed (Favre et al. 2006). The less adapted and immature defense mechanisms, such as projection or denial, globally decreased after CST, while the general defensive level improved. We concluded that a wide variety of defense mechanisms are operant in oncology clinicians facing challenging interviews, and that defense mechanisms may be modified by CST

(Favre et al. 2006). Since these results could partially answer the question of how CST works, a more comprehensive and controlled study is currently conducted.

11.7   Conclusions

A review of the scientific literature on CST in oncology reveals a fascinating field of research, most relevant for oncology practice. While evidence exists that these training sessions induce change toward more patient-centered communication, several methodological difficulties associated with these studies persist. Most important, a variety of confounding variables exist, and there is a lack of understanding of how CST induces change. Despite the fact that the participant himself is probably the most important variable of variance in outcome, none of the published studies has investigated this topic to date. Research on medical communication and CST is only emerging. Hopefully, the clinician caring for patients will increasingly become a topic of interest and scientific investigation. Practicing medicine implies the encounter between (at least) two persons, namely the patient and the clinician; it is rather curious that up to now the overwhelming majority of scientific efforts of medical psychology has only focused on the patient.

References

1. Booth K, Maguire P (1991) Cancer research campaign interview rating manual. Alphabet Studio, Manchester
2. Fallowfield L (1995) Can we improve the professional and personal fulfilment of doctors in cancer medicine? Br J Cancer 71:1132–1133
3. Fallowfield L, Jenkins V, Farewell V, Saul J, Duffy A, Eves R (2002) Efficacy of a cancer research UK communication skills training model for oncologists: a randomised controlled trial. Lancet 359:650–656
4. Fallowfield L, Jenkins V, Farewell V, Solis-Trapala I (2003) Enduring impact of communication skills training: results of a 12-month follow-up. Br J Cancer 89:1445–1449
5. Faulkner A, Argent J, Jones A, O'Keeffe C (1995) Improving the skills of doctors in giving distressing information. Med Educ 29:303–307
6. Favre N, Despland J-N, de Rothen Y, et al (2006) Psychodynamic aspects of communication skills training in oncology: pilot study. (submitted)
7. Fellowes D, Wilkinson S, Moore P (2004) Communication skills training for health care professionals working with cancer patients, their families and/or carers. Cochrane Database Syst Rev 2004:CD003751
8. Fitzgerald A, Mayrhofer D, Huber R, Fitzgerarld RD (2004) The COPe concept for the training of communication in highly emotional situations. Ann Transplant 9:36–38
9. Ford S, Fallowfield L, Lewis S (1996) Doctor-patient interactions in oncology. Soc Sci Med 42:1511–1519
10. Ford S, Hall A, Ratcliffe D, Fallowfield L (2000) The Medical Interaction Process System (MIPS): an instrument for analysing interviews of oncologists and patients with cancer. Soc Sci Med 50:553–566
11. Guex P, Stiefel F, Rousselle I (2002) La communication: un élément central en cancérologie. Rev Francoph Psycho-Oncol 1:43–46
12. Gysels M, Richardson A, Higginson IJ (2004) Communication training for health professionals who care for patients with cancer: a systematic review of effectiveness. Support Care Cancer 12:692–700
13. Gysels M, Richardson A, Higginson IJ (2005) Communication training for health professionals who care for patients with cancer: a systematic review of training methods. Support Care Cancer 13:356–366
14. Hürny C (2000) Communiquer, ce n'est pas un choix. Bull Suisse Cancer 1:1–2
15. Jenkins V, Fallowfield L (2002) Can communication skills training alter physicians' beliefs and behavior in clinics? J Clin Oncol 20:765–769
16. Klein S (1999) The effects of the participation of patients with cancer in teaching communication skills to medical undergraduates: a randomized study with follow-up after 2 years. Eur J Cancer 35:1448–1456
17. Lerman C, Daly M, Walsh WP, Resch N, Seay J, Barsevick A, Birenbaum L, Heggan T, Martin G (1993) Communication between patients with breast cancer and health care providers: determinants and implications. Cancer 72:2612–2620

18. Loge JH, Kaasa S, Hytten K (1997) Disclosing the cancer diagnosis: the patients' experiences. Eur J Cancer 33:878–882

19. Maguire P, Booth K, Elliott C, Jones B (1996) Helping health professionals involved in cancer care acquire key interviewing skills—the impact of workshops. Eur J Cancer 32A:1486–1489

20. Ong LM, de Haes JC, Hoos AM, Lammes FB (1995) Doctor-patient communication: a review of the literature. Soc Sci Med 40:903–918

21. Ong LM, Visse MR, Lammes FB, de Haes JC (2000) Doctor-patient communication and cancer patient's quality of life and satisfaction. Patient Couns Health Educ 41:145–156

22. Perry JC (1990) Defense mechanism rating scale, 5th edn. Cambridge University, Boston

23. Perry JC, Cooper S (1989) An empirical study of defense mechanisms. Arch Gen Psychiatry 46:444–452

24. Ramirez AJ, Graham J, Richards MA, Cull A, Gregory WM (1996) Mental health of hospital consultants: the effects of stress and satisfaction at work. Lancet 347:724–728

25. Razavi D, Delvaux N, Marchal S, De Cock M, Farvacques C, Slachmuylder JL (2000) Testing health care professionals' communication skills: the usefulness of highly emotional standardized role-playing sessions with simulators. Psychooncology 9:293–302

26. Razavi D, Merckaert I, Marchal S, Libert Y, Conradt S, Boniver J, Etienne AM, Fontaine O, Janne P, Klastersky J, Reynaert C, Scalliet P, Slachmuylder JL, Delvaux N (2003) How to optimize physicians' communication skills in cancer care: results of a randomized study assessing the usefulness of posttraining consolidation workshops. J Clin Oncol 21:3141–3149

27. Wilkinson S (1991) Factors which influence how nurses communicate with cancer patients. J Adv Nurs 16:677–688

28. Wilkinson S, Roberts A, Aldridge J (1998) Nurse-patient communication in palliative care: an evaluation of a communication skills programme. Palliat Med 12:13–22

29. Wilkinson S, Bailey K, Aldridge J, Roberts A (1999) A longitudinal evaluation of a communication skills programme. Palliat Med 13:341–348

30. Wilkinson SM, Gambles M, Roberts A (2002) The essence of cancer care: the impact of training on nurses' ability to communicate effectively. J Adv Nurs 40:731–738

12 Communication and Communication Skills Training in Oncology: Open Questions and Future Tasks

A. Kiss, W. Söllner

Recent Results in Cancer Research, Vol. 168
© Springer-Verlag Berlin Heidelberg 2006

Summary

Based on their experience as teachers of communication skills training for oncology clinicians, the authors report their observations and reflect on open questions and future challenges with regard to communication in cancer care.

Both of us have been training oncologists and oncology nurses in communication skills training (CST) for many years (Kiss 1999). This might be the reason why the editor asked us to comment on CST from a clinical point of view. We will therefore share some observations we made while doing such training and we will try to define future tasks.

12.1 The Gap Between Research and Practice

At first glance, CST in oncology seems to be a success story. The effectiveness of such training has been demonstrated by a randomised trial with UK oncologists (Fallowfield et al. 2002). Research in patient–professional communication in cancer is growing, as illustrated by the fact that a special issue of the journal Psycho-Oncology has been devoted to this subject (Hack 2005) and that the results of communication skills training are published in mainstream cancer journals (Delvaux et al. 2005). CST that focuses on specific topics such as shared decision-making, detecting psychosocial distress in cancer patients and information about randomised clinical trials has been developed and evaluated recently (Jenkins et al. 2005). Finally, communication skills training has become mandatory in some curricula in oncology and haematology.

However, some open questions remain concerning how to translate the results of this research into clinical practice:

1. Who will pay for the CST if it becomes part of the training of oncologists and oncology nurses? Effective training has to be conducted in small groups, with an experienced trainer, which is costly. Resources for continuing medical education (CME) are limited, and sponsorships from pharmaceutical companies have become difficult. Our experience in Switzerland, Austria and Germany is that physicians are able to pay themselves, but nurses can hardly afford it. In recent years, the support of hospitals for working leaves and funding has diminished.

2. To the best of our knowledge almost all randomised trials of CST in oncology were conducted with participants who volunteered. For example, in the study of Merckaert and co-workers (2005), the final sample of 72 participants was based on 214 invitations to participate made by telephone, 163 individuals were informed personally and 173 in groups. This means that the participants were probably highly motivated and not representative. If the aim of CST is not only to "preach to the converted" but also to include a larger group, we do not know if the effect of the training will be the same. Our experience in Switzerland, where CST is mandatory for oncologists, is that most physicians appreciate the train-

ing, but some do not and the improvement of their communication skills may therefore be moderate.

3. Until now, most training has been provided by very motivated and enthusiastic trainers who have worked in this field for years. If CST is to spread, more trainers will be needed. To form these trainers, "train the trainer courses" will be necessary. Whether or not these new trainers will be as effective as the current ones is unknown.

4. Outcome measurements such as analysis of the communication of professionals interacting with simulated or real patients before and after training is costly and time consuming, and experienced raters are needed. How can quality of future training be assessed while funding is restricted? It is unclear what kind of measurement is appropriate to evaluate such training. Maybe rating tools that assess communication competence could serve to measure outcomes in a less costly way (Schirmer et al. 2005).

12.2 Why Is CST a Major Theme Only in Oncology?

It is hard to find any scientific literature on CST in other specialities, e.g. gastroenterology or cardiology. In gastroenterology the most frequent patients are those with functional disorders such as irritable bowel syndrome. Until now, no trial has been effectuated to demonstrate that a CST enhances communication competence of gastroenterologists (Drossman 2005). To give another example: Severe chronic heart failure has a worse prognosis than many malignancies. However, we are not aware of any CST of cardiologists, who often have to give bad news to patients and inform them about their prognosis.

One major reason may be that oncology is still linked with the image of incurable and suffering patients, despite the fact that nowadays about half of all cancer patients can be cured. There seems to be a change in current attitude: The Institute of Medicine in its 2004 report, "Improving Medical Education: Enhancing the Behavioral and Social Science Content of Medical School Curricula" identifies communication skills as one of six curricular domains (Institute of Medicine 2004). CST in oncology is a first step; other specialities will follow.

12.3 Do We Contribute to the Strain of Healthcare Providers in Palliative Care?

Poor communication with patients and their relatives may be a consequence of unresolved distress of healthcare providers, but it may also constitute a source of major distress in physicians and nurses providing palliative care (Simpson et al. 1991). However, adequate communication with the severely ill and the dying patient and his loved ones may also cause distress and—if coping mechanisms fail—burnout. The desire to be a good caregiver who not only provides efficient, good medical treatment but also does her best to adequately communicate and to emotionally support the patient and his family may overburden the clinician. Palliative care is characterised by close and caring relationships and emotionally intensive work on the one hand, and anxiety and anger arising from the repeated confrontation with death and dying, on the other. This requires adequate coping strategies and balanced relationship between proximity and distance with the patient (Kash and Holland 1990). Distancing oneself from patients and their suffering and concentrating on medically routine tasks are self-protective behaviours. If confronted with multiple stressors while lacking adequate coping strategies like seeking self-esteem in interests other than caring for patients (work–life balance) or mobilising support from colleagues and friends, distancing oneself from patients may last and become a symptom of burnout (Lown 1996; Lopez-Castillo et al. 1999; Maslach et al. 2001).

The demands of better understanding and meeting the psychosocial needs of the severely ill may further increase feelings of insufficiency and failure in healthcare providers who fail to adequately distance themselves from the suffering of their patients. As a consequence, those who provide CST—especially if it is mandatory—should always take into account the trainees' resilence and their skills at coping with repeated bereavements. In our opinion, training should include small-group discussions of the trainees' work-related emotional distress and their coping strategies. Rigid and straining demands on oneself often arise from an unconscious wish to "heal" severely ill patients rather than to accompany and care for them in their last period of life. Such motivations should be addressed and analysed. Trainees should not be confronted with new demands like better communication behaviour with patients and their loved ones without reducing such overtaxing demands to the self. Our experience in guiding CST led us to combine such training with a limited and work-related process of self-reflection and self-experience (Balint 1964). We learned by experience that participation in theme-centred small-group discussions or Balint groups opens a space of reflection and allows participants to decrease unrealistic self-demands and to improve self-protective behaviours. Often this is a prerequisite for an effective CST.

12.4 Why Is the Focus Only on the Patient, While Communication Within the Healthcare System Is Often Neglected?

Severely and chronically ill patients often complain about poor communication between medical specialists and between physicians and nurses in the hospital, as well as poor communication between specialists and family physicians. Poor communication leads to unclear and often conflicting information on patients and their relatives, and subsequent uncertainty, ambivalence and sometimes difficulty in complying with treatment. Quality management and organisational development activities can address horizontal (inside the hospital) or vertical (between hospital and ambulatory care) communication problems within the healthcare system, can analyse the reasons for them and develop solutions (Schaufeli and Enzmann 1998).

Better communication within the hospital is impeded by recent developments such as the re-

ducing length of stay in hospitals without adjusting the offer of ambulatory care, staff shortening in oncological or palliative care units, cutting reimbursement and "outsourcing" of psycho-social services. These factors prevent trainees who successfully take part in a communication skills course from putting their new knowledge and skills into clinical practice. Such frustrating experiences may lead to resignation and a relapse to "old" communication patterns. CST on an individual level should be accompanied by efforts on a systemic level to develop adequate conditions for better communication. This includes quality management activities as well as political commitment.

12.5 What Does It Take to Become a Good Trainer for CST in Oncology?

CST will spread, since communication has been recognised as a key element of cancer care; therefore, it is worth identify the qualifications of a good trainer.

12.5.1 Personality

Trainers should be comfortable and enjoy communication with other people. They should have a talent for dealing with unexpected situations and the ability to focus more on persons' resources than on their shortcomings. Trainers should be reflective and open-minded about processes of work-related self-experience. To decrease the risks of the development of pressure towards perfectionism and of developing burnout in the trainees, trainers should acknowledge their own limits and abstain from promoting narcissistic feelings in the trainees ("becoming a perfect physician/nurse").

12.5.2 Professional Background

Most trainers are either healthcare professionals or clinical psychologists. Both backgrounds have their advantages and disadvantages: Healthcare professionals are more familiar with the medical environment but tend to underestimate that changing human behaviour, i.e. communicating in a different way, is a very complex and challenging task. Clinical psychologists on the other hand tend to underestimate the specifics of medicine because they are not familiar with this work. In our experience, working in a psychiatric or psychosomatic consultation-liaison service in a palliative care or oncology unit and therefore being familiar with the demands and problems of this kind of work is a good prerequisite for becoming a trainer (Breitbart and Lintz 2002; Söllner et al. 2004). Regardless of the professional background, trainers should be familiar with group dynamics. They should be able to provide a protective and supportive environment in the group that allows each trainee to openly address his problems of communication with severely ill and dying patients.

12.5.3 Framework

In order to teach communication skills, a multidimensional framework is needed. A learner-centred approach is essential:
The essential characteristics are provision of a cognitive component or evidence base for suggested skills, a behavioural component allowing participants to rehearse the actual communication skills required through role play with patient actors playing patients, and an affective component permitting participants to explore the feelings that communicating about difficult issues evoke (Fallowfield and Jenkins 2004).

12.5.4 Supervision

The first step should be that future trainers participate themselves in a CST as a trainee. Then, specific parts of the training should be done by future trainers under supervision of experienced trainers. The easiest part involves the lectures; the most difficult involves the interactions such as role-playing, giving feedback and dealing with group dynamics. As it is currently demanded from trainee doctors and nurses that they videotape interaction with simulated or real patients,

it should be the same for future trainers to videotape themselves when they interact with participants of CST.

Communication in cancer care has been recognised as an important task in the daily clinical oncology practice, and the first steps towards improving the communication skills of oncology clinicians have been undertaken. A wider implementation of CST in oncology faces various challenges and obstacles. As with any other medical activity, progress in communication will require a comprehensive reflection of the topic, courageous and skillful trainers who are able to "spread the message" and a rigorous scientific investigation to accompany these efforts.

References

1. Balint M (1964) The doctor, his patient, and the illness. Pitman Medical Publishing, London
2. Breitbart W, Lintz K (2002) Psychiatric issues in the care of dying patients. In: Wise MG, Rundell JR (eds) Textbook of consultation—liaison psychiatry. The American Psychiatric Publishing, London, pp 771–804
3. Delvaux N, Merckaert I, Marchal S, Libert Y, Conradt S, Boniver J, Etienne AM, Fontaine O, Janne P, Klastersky J, Melot C, Reynaert C, Scalliet P, Slachmuylder JL, Razavi D (2005) Physicians' communication with a cancer patient and a relative: a randomized study assessing the efficacy of consolidation workshops. Cancer 103:2397–2411
4. Drossman DA (2005) What does the future hold for irritable bowel syndrome and the functional gastrointestinal disorders? J Clin Gastroenterol 39:S251–S256
5. Fallowfield L, Jenkins V (2004) Communicating sad, bad, and difficult news in medicine. Lancet 363:312–319
6. Fallowfield L, Jenkins V, Farewell V, Saul J, Duffy A, Eves R (2002) Efficacy of a Cancer Research UK communication skills training model for oncologists: a randomised controlled trial. Lancet 359:650–656
7. Hack T (2005) Psycho-oncology special issue on communication. Psychooncology 14:797–798
8. Institute of Medicine (2004) Improving medical education. Enhancing the behavioral and social science content of medical school curricula. The National Academic Press, Washington

9. Jenkins V, Fallowfield L, Solis-Trapala I, Langridge C, Farewell V (2005) Discussing randomised clinical trials of cancer therapy: evaluation of a Cancer Research UK training programme. BMJ 330:400

10. Kash KM, Holland JC (1990) Reducing stress in medical oncology house officers: a preliminary report of a prospective intervention study. In: Hendrie HC, Lloyd C, Roeske NA (eds) Educating competent and humane physicians. Indiana University Press, Bloomington, pp 183–195

11. Kiss A (1999) Communication skills training in oncology: a position paper. Ann Oncol 10:899–901

12. Lopez-Castillo J, Gurpegui M, Ayuso-Mateos JL, Luna JD, Catalan J (1999) Emotional distress and occupational burnout in health care professionals serving HIV-infected patients: a comparison with oncology and internal medicine services. Psychother Psychosom 68:348–356

13. Lown B (1996) The lost art of healing. Ballantine Books, New York

14. Maslach C, Schaufeli WB, Leiter MP (2001) Job burnout. Annu Rev Psychol 52:397–422

15. Merckaert I, Libert Y, Delvaux N, Marchal S, Boniver J, Etienne AM, Klastersky J, Reynaert C, Scalliet P, Slachmuylder JL, Razavi D (2005) Factors that influence physicians' detection of distress in patients with cancer: can a communication skills training program improve physicians' detection? Cancer 104:411–421

16. Schaufeli WB, Enzmann D (1998) The burnout companion to study and practice. Taylor and Francis, London

17. Schirmer JM, Mauksch L, Lang F, Marvel MK, Zoppi K, Epstein RM, Brock D, Pryzbylski M (2005) Assessing communication competence: a review of current tools. Fam Med 37:184–192

18. Simpson M, Buckman R, Stewart M, Maguire P, Lipkin M, Novack D, Till J (1991) Doctor-patient communication: the Toronto consensus statement. BMJ 303:1385–1387

19. Söllner W, Maislinger S, König A, DeVries A, Lukas P (2004) Providing psychosocial support for breast cancer patients based on screening for distress within a consultation-liaison service. Psychooncology 13:893–897